The Dizzy Woman's Bathtub Guide

The Dizzy Woman's Bathtub Guide

Exercises for a Balanced Body

Suzanne Kay, PT

Illustrated by Jose Sandoval & Gina Kay

TATE PUBLISHING
AND ENTERPRISES, LLC

The Dizzy Woman's Bathtub Guide
Copyright © 2015 by Suzanne Kay, PT. All rights reserved.

No part of this publication may be reproduced, stored in a retrieval system or transmitted in any way by any means, electronic, mechanical, photocopy, recording or otherwise without the prior permission of the author except as provided by USA copyright law.

The opinions expressed by the author are not necessarily those of Tate Publishing, LLC.

Published by Tate Publishing & Enterprises, LLC
127 E. Trade Center Terrace | Mustang, Oklahoma 73064 USA
1.888.361.9473 | www.tatepublishing.com

Tate Publishing is committed to excellence in the publishing industry. The company reflects the philosophy established by the founders, based on Psalm 68:11,
"The Lord gave the word and great was the company of those who published it."

Book design copyright © 2015 by Tate Publishing, LLC. All rights reserved.
Cover design by Joseph Emnace
Interior design by Gram Telen
Illustrations by Jose Sandoval and Gina Kay

Published in the United States of America

ISBN: 978-1-63268-660-2
1. Self-Help / Healthy Living
2. Health & Fitness / Women's Health
15.04.13

This book is dedicated to My Mom,
for being a wonderful example
to me through my life
on the importance of balancing family and career,
generosity and frugalness,
determination and realism,
acceptance and courage.
I love you Mom.

Acknowledgments

There are so many people that have taught and inspired me over the years and helped to bring me to the point of producing this book: teachers, co-workers, patients, counselors, spiritual leaders, authors, family, friends, musicians. It is amazing how even people we may not know personally can impact our life journey. There are some whom I would like to acknowledge individually of course. First off, I could not have shared this book if it were not for all the skilled professionals at Tate Publishing, especially Stacy Baker, who believed in this project from the beginning and Erin Vaught and Eden Pancho who supported this first time author through the world of editing and publishing. I must also thank my pastor, Father Jorge Hernandez, who spoke words of faith and healing to help me believe in God's perfect timing in bringing this book to fruition. Much thanks to my old friend Chris Lewis who helped me feel confident and joyfully captured my spirit from behind his lens. To my special friends who held my hand through some of the most painful years of my life and then cheered me on while I found my voice again and learned to share it- "The Peacocks": Laura Paule, Sally Moncrieff, Laurel Jamtgaard and Kristi Norton, Ann-Marie Cordova, Tony DeSilva, Diane Wells, Corrine Smith, Tammy West and Christine Zetterberg–you are forever friends and I am blessed to have you in my life. To my mom, who first planted the seed, many years prior, saying "You could write," believing in me despite my limitations. To my dad whose hearty laugh helped me develop the title and theme of my modest book. To my precious children, Gina, my personal illustrator extraordinaire; and Ian and Anna, my computer consultants and public relations experts, thank you for accepting your mom is not a perfect parent, but has a perfect love for each of you. And to my husband Tim of over twenty years- my first and forever love- thank you for all the extra loads of laundry and dishes you so patiently did without any complaints while I completed this book, spending much more time on the computer or in the bathtub than the average wife. Average is definitely not the word for all the people mentioned above... the word that comes to mind is exceptional, and I love and am grateful for all of you!

Contents

Introduction 11
The Beauty of the Bath 17
Bathing for Beginners 37
Stretch Yourself 49
Upper Body Urgency 65
The Power's in the Legs 83
Tummy Time 104
Shower Sequel 127
Finally the Feat 137
Quick Position Guide to Exercise Sequence 145

Introduction

I can now get up and down my stairs without feeling twenty years older than I actually am. I may not be able to run a marathon anymore, but I can certainly cross a finish line in a multiplicity of life events without hitting the wall. I can laugh at myself. I can love myself scars and all. I am confident enough to believe in myself even when others may not. I can acknowledge both my strengths and weaknesses while attempting to actively strengthen both. No longer do I psychologically punish myself every time I make a silly mistake like dropping my phone in the toilet or misplacing my car keys. I no longer look at everything that goes "wrong" in my life as somehow being my fault.

For years however, I could not have honestly made the above statements. I struggled daily with the balancing act of life. The deeper I got into the ranks of middle age, the more out of sync I felt and the more depressed and anxious I became as I repeatedly suffered from a variety of physical ailments.

I loved my work, but I couldn't handle the physical and emotional demands of my job. I loved my God, but I wallowed in guilt and shame and constantly felt I was falling short of meeting what I perceived were his expectations of me. I loved my children, but I was overwhelmed and overly critical of my parenting skills.

It took some deep soul searching during a barrage of personal life struggles to begin to understand some essential elements to turn my life around and begin to lead a better balanced life. During my search for well being I was drawn to God's word. Therein I found love to be the main theme of the bible. Jesus said to love others as I have loved you and to love others as you love yourself. Therefore it follows that in order to love others fully, one must be open to God's unconditional love as well as love oneself in such a way.

Coming from a traditional Christian background, my paradigm may be different than yours. As our faith calls us to evangelize, I would be delighted if this book spurs you to explore Christianity at a deeper level. However, I do not in anyway intend to disrespect your belief system. We all can learn from one another by being peacefully open-minded and nonjudgmental. Please try to take what you can from my point of view and make it your own. Spirituality, just as growth in body and mind, is an individual's personal journey and one that can take many different roads to eventually mysteriously end in the same beautiful place of truth and love.

Health and healing work in much the same manner. In order to live a healthy, functional life, I believe one must accept three basic principles. First, God is the master healer. Second, God often works his miracles through the disguise of others who are open to his love and grace. Thirdly, one must accept that God places inside each one of us the amazing ability to heal ourselves if we are truly open to all the gifts he wants to share as he dwells within us.

It was through balancing these three principles in my self imposed tumultuous life, that as I dealt with the physical issues I was having, I simultaneously began to heal the emotional wounds that had been growing inside me since my childhood. I then became free to begin experiencing the life I was meant to live. A life balanced with peace, joy, faith, health, hope and love had eluded me for years until I discovered the practical exercises (both physical and mental) explained in this book. I certainly had much love in my life, although I had often misconstrued that I was more on the giving than the receiving end. I had periods of joy, but they tended to be fleeting and often replaced by despair. Although often called a dreamer, true hope was usually absent . Peace nearly always eluded me.

God put many people in my life—therapists, counselors, doctors, psychologists, teachers, clergy, patients, family and friends who helped me along my road of healing. But I had to take the steps. I had to do the hard work of being truthful with, patient with, persistent with, and forgiving of myself to reach my end goal of physical and emotional health. I had to learn from information gained and follow the sound advice offered.

I discovered too, that there really is never an end to such a process. There are still areas of my life I need to work on. I will always strive to improve myself and become wiser, stronger, and healthier physically, emotionally, and spiritually. I know I will never reach perfection- not until I meet my Maker and he deems me passage into his world. But in the meantime, I will continue to strive toward enjoying this gift called life with a positive attitude and a peaceful spirit. I know that life will continue to offer countless challenging opportunities to test my positive, peaceful, balanced body, mind and spirit. But practice makes progress!

I realize now we are all essentially made perfect through our imperfections. They are what make us unique children of God who must turn to him for support and guidance. Whether I am feeling lost and floundering or when things seems to be heading in the right direction, I know as long as I am allowing God to guide me, I can be at peace in the moment, no matter what the circumstances. I can draw upon him for the strength needed both physically, spiritually and emotionally to get through any struggle.

This book is my attempt to help others prepare to deal with physical and or emotional pain in a positive and proactive way. As a physical therapist I have sat in the back seat to hundreds if not thousands of people's pain and suffering. Ironically, although I believe I have been able to help many people, once

I sat in the drivers seat, I initially had a hard time helping myself. I believe my experiences have been a gift to help me learn much more about what it really means to find health and healing. I hope to share the knowledge and wisdom I have gained over the past twenty five years of my career and life to help others. I may not be able to lay on my hands or share a smile, but I can still offer words of encouragement and hope for the future.

In all humility, the credit for this book and any help one may receive from it goes to God and God alone. He is the inspiration behind putting all this to words. He is the soul of this book. I never would have thrived or even survived my past five years, or my entire life for that matter without His amazing grace and constant presence. He is after all the master healer.

The Beauty of the Bath

Being a busy woman is one thing. Being a *dizzy* woman is something else. I am not referring to the *dizzy blond* stereotype of old. Many of the most intelligent and powerful woman I know are blonds and large numbers of women who don't sport blond locks pay for an expensive dye job to attain that image. Most of us females are busy. It's just the reality of the society we live in and the expectations set upon us.

Rarely will you find the fantasy woman who sits around all day eating chocolate truffles and texting friends while watching the latest reality show episode. If that woman is out there, then her life is out of balance in a different way, and it's time to get a little more active.

The dizzy woman, however—this is totally different. This is busyness to the point that your world is spinning and you can't achieve focus. We've all had moments of this feeling, but when one begins to feel out of balance the majority of the time, there is an issue. If crashing and falling from the vertigo of life begins to be a danger that you anticipate with fear and trepidation on a daily basis, then this book will be a godsend to you. But even the most put-together woman, if she is honest with herself, has areas of her life that are out of balance.

Balance is not something that once attained is maintained with ease. Constant readjustment to the unexpected challenges of life requires strength, flexibility, and grace. If one of those components are compromised, then it takes some work to make quality balance even possible. Even with an out-of-whack system, one can achieve precarious balance, but it can be exhausting and even painful. If there are not issues currently, then eventually, when the load becomes too heavy, there most likely will be.

This book is about gaining the balance needed to not only function in life, but to enjoy the journey. Our body is the transportation on our journey. We cannot exchange our bodies for a newer model when we blow a gasket or things start to go wrong. Rebuilding the engine is possible, but good maintenance is much less expensive and much less painful.

No matter what you are striving for—more time for your family, more time for yourself, a healthier lifestyle, weight loss, chronic pain alleviation, career advancement, financial freedom—whatever your life goals, if you are having difficulty achieving them or if you are overachieving to the point of neglecting other areas of your life, this book can help you to put your life balance into perspective. Before we can tackle exterior goals however, we need to look within our own microcosm, which is our body's environment. Before you can achieve peace and beauty in your exterior world, one needs to focus on creating beauty and balance interiorly.

A beautiful body by our world's definition is something that most women dream of, but few attain. The few that do attain the goal frequently have trouble retaining it! The reason that this is such a challenge is that most of us have the definition confused. In my opinion, it is the process of improving ourselves—both body and soul—that is beautiful. Let us focus on relishing each precious moment of progress that has been made so that we feel better today than yesterday, even if it is just in some small way.

The definition of a beautifully balanced body doesn't mean a thinner body or a body with cut-muscle definition. A beautiful body means a body that feels and performs better—physically, emotionally, and mentally. A balanced body is one that has the energy you need when you need it, has the strength and flexibility you need when you need it, and has the stamina you need when you need it—emotionally, intellectually, and physically to lead the life you were meant to live. Our body, mind, and spirit create a dynamic system that works together, hopefully in harmony. You cannot neglect one area and expect another area to take up the slack. That is not how we were designed. My goal is that in the perusing of this book, you will relax and work, laugh and cry, plan and reflect, read and imagine, and learn to love your body, and hence, love yourself.

When we have a thing of beauty, we should honor it. A gorgeous painting is not stuck in a dark hallway held up by a tack. A frame to give structure, glass for protection, and a matte to accentuate the vibrant colors, attaches the artwork to the wall with a good sturdy mount. So too should we develop a good musculoskeletal system for structure and protection. We should adorn our bodies with colors that set off our natural beauty and lotions that cleanse and soften our skin as well as tantalize the olfactory system. Although not visible to the viewer, what's within the framework is the food we feed our bodies and souls. Many of us think about the food we eat and the fluids we drink as nourishment to our body. However, the books we read, the movies we watch, the internet sites we frequently visit, and the music we listen to are all examples of the food we feed our mind and souls.

Most of us have experienced how the positive energy that certain people exude makes us feel more energetic, more motivated, or more loved. Unfortunately, on the negative side, there are also those certain people that just have a dimming effect on the psyche. A dear friend of mine refers to such people as "emotional vampires" or "joy suckers". Protect yourself from such people, and by all means, do not be one! The trick is learning how to create positive energy within yourself. There is a scientific principle called the Krebs cycle that proves one basic phenomena—movement creates energy! This does not mean you need to run ten miles a day or go to a kickboxing class for ninety minutes. That is just not a lot of people's idea of a good time nor is it necessary to have a beautiful balance between body and spirit. Everyone should be able to find a dynamic activity that is both enjoyable and healthy to create the positive energy that is so needed in a healthy life. Bathing has not typically been thought of as a very dynamic activity, rather the opposite- a relaxing activity. The beauty is that it can be both!

Life is all about balance. Balancing counteracting muscle groups for good posture, balancing work and play for a healthy lifestyle, balancing self-sacrifice with self-care for viable relationships—the list is endless. Ironically, my senior seminar in physical therapy school was on balance. The reason that is an irony, is that although balance was always at the core of my treatment plans to help bring others to health and function in their life, it took me about twenty years after graduation from one of the most esteemed medical institutions in the country, to finally understand the true meaning of balance in my own life.

Understanding a problem is just the beginning of solving it, however. After identifying the lack of balance in my own life, it has been a daily process to seek balance. Balance is something your body and mind must coordinate on an ongoing basis, virtually every waking moment. At times we will falter, we will stagger, we will wobble and work so hard to not fall off that balance beam called life. Days will come when we stumble and jump up uninjured. Other times, a misstep which seems minor can result in a major issue.

Recovery from the inevitable minor or major injuries of life, be they from random events or poor balance, is reliant on both our physical and spiritual strength. God supplies the spiritual strength, and we need to do our part when it comes to the physical conditioning. How long it takes to get your bearings is to a large extent reliant on how healthy you are at baseline and how much attention you pay to nurturing day to day balance in your life.

There may be moments, days, even weeks that get out of balance through no fault of one's own. But if you rebalance yourself regularly by taking prayerful time to figure out what is causing the scales to tip, then do the necessary work to restructure your life, equilibrium can always be found again. Lots of introspection and a day-to-day regrouping of priorities is a necessary task for me to maintain balance in my own life. Each day different challenges, circumstances, pleasures, and priorities can tip the scales in one direction or another. As long as you don't bottom out the scale, you're doing fine. For quite some time, I had to put a picture on my bathroom mirror of a scale to remind me to keep my day and hence my life in balance.

P_____P
▲

I'll explain the details of my scale later.

The focus of this book is balancing strength, flexibility, relaxation and activity. Although an extremely important exercise tool and one that should be factored in as a component in having a healthy, balanced lifestyle, endurance is not really the focus of this book. Since aerobic activity is a huge factor is calorie consumption, there are no guarantees this book will change you from a size sixteen to a size eight. Personally, my weight fluctuates quite a bit due to the season of life I am in.

Although many charts and online sources will tell you a woman of five feet six inches ideally should weigh below 150 pounds, I must admit I do not currently fall into that category. Although I may get there again someday, I believe it is more important to get to know and love yourself and your body and not over focus on weight loss goals. If one truly loves themselves, being good to oneself will come more easily as will any necessary weight loss that may be needed. Pounds do not necessarily reflect health. Being on the more curvy side personally, I would like to think I have more muscles than the average pushing fifty year old. Also, I think I need a little extra umph behind me when I am coercing sometimes 200-plus-pound patients out of a hospital bed and into a wheelchair or onto a walker, or lifting a child with cerebral palsy out of her wheelchair and onto the mat for her morning warm-up. It's commonly known that muscle weighs more than fat. And of course, I am as well hopeful that there is not much empty air space in my bones—"Just say no to osteo" (porosis, that is).

The adage that the scale doesn't lie is a lie. BMI (body mass index), the more recent tool used to assure that your height-to-weight ratio is a healthy one, can also be deceiving. Using the BMI as an indicator for healthy weight is not always accurate for people who have more inches or more muscle than the average individual. It also does not take into account your proportions. More recent research is showing that individuals who carry more of their extra pounds on their hips have less health issues than those who carry extra weight in their midriff.

Maybe when I was a premenopausal adult female, a lofty weight loss goal would have been realistic for me. However, I wouldn't want to go back to the body image and self-esteem that I had in my young adult years. I must tell you though, that the Wii Fit put me at twenty-nine Wii age recently and I was quite tickled! Prior to starting my bathtub program, which I developed basically because I wanted to have what I call justified relaxation time, I was struggling significantly with generalized aches and pains. Granted, I know we should not have to justify relaxing, but unfortunately that is the reality of the mindset situation for many women in today's world. Becoming my own version of a bathing beauty, I slowly began to feel better as I focused on nurturing both my body and my spirit, while I simultaneously got squeaky clean. The point I am trying to make is to not get too hung up on how much you weigh, but focus instead on how you feel and think positive thoughts about yourself, even if at first you feel like you are making justifications.

Early on, my chronic pain issues were blamed on depression—who wouldn't be depressed I ask you when you feel lousy most of the time? Synonymous to "What came first, the chicken or the egg?" was the question, "What came first, the depression or the pain?" It was a question I was constantly trying to figure out. Having a history of being a competitive runner and an outdoors woman, as I eked past forty, I became more and more limited in my ability to participate in activities I loved. I jokingly told friends and colleagues that I suffered from crappy cartilage syndrome (early arthritis). Being very in tune to my body, I noticed every ache and pain like a determined kid finds pictures in an *I Spy* book. These aches and pains weren't necessary to alert my body to some danger, they were just the signs of change. And needless to say, as I entered the ranks of single motherhood after seventeen years of marriage, my anxiety about that changing body and how I could continue doing my physically demanding work was extremely heightened.

However that anxiety eventually contributed to the development of some major issues in my life. On top of the dull, aching, generalized pain, I had become used to, I began intermittently experiencing numbness and tingling in my hands and feet and even more disturbingly in my left arm, which was exacerbated when I was using my arm to support a patient. I was fearful that I might suddenly lose strength and a patient could be hurt and felt for everyone's safety I needed to take some time off work. Since I had just begun a new job after shutting down my private practice when these issues began, I had not hit the six-month probationary period when I informed my employer of my situation. What exactly the issue was remained unclear. Two different MRIs showed two different possibilities. Degenerative disk disease and arthritis in my neck was the most likely explanation, but I also had lesions in my central nervous system that could be indicators of multiple sclerosis (MS). Thankfully, other tests however did not support the diagnosis of MS.

I mistakenly thought I would be met by compassion and accommodations by my employer, especially being in the rehabilitation field. Unfortunately, a four-week leave of absence due to physical and mental health issues did not mesh well with the beginning of the post-George W. Bush economic crisis.

Shortly after returning from my medical leave, my "Probationary employment was not extended." Although I initially was quite angry with what I thought was an injustice, in retrospect I have to admit that the timing was right to experience my first ever bout with unemployment. I was able to be home during the summer with my kids and had more time to help them and myself adjust to the two-household lifestyle and the idea that a nuclear family was not necessarily a healthy one as far as our situation was concerned at that time.

I also had time that summer to discover the haven of my bathtub. My eldest daughter always loved her bath, even as a teenager. I rarely used the tub unless she was at her Dad's and then after she left both our homes, which unfortunately was not on the most peaceful of terms. Losing my eldest daughter, or what I perceived at the time as losing her, when in effect, it was only a temporary misplacement, was just as difficult for me as the demise of my marriage. It was during this time that I turned to my bathtub for support; and as a byproduct of that this book was conceived and born.

I began the healing process both physically and emotionally that summer and moved forward. It was a time of great dichotomy. I experienced some of the greatest grief and joy of my life. I experienced both atrocious anxiety and profound peace. I experienced being on the receiving end instead of the giving end, when I had to get a food box from my church and put my kids on the free and reduced lunch program at their schools. It was a humbling experience to say the least, but one that I would not trade for the world.

These experiences were part of my journey toward being the woman God intended me to be. I truly believe that any bad situation can be turned into good if you sincerely ask for Divine help and guidance and trust that although you may not understand, agree with, or enjoy the process of change, God knows what is best for you and loves you beyond comprehension.

I had so many preconceived notions change that summer. I sadly realized I had passed judgments on a multiplicity of people in different and difficult situations in the past, be it homelessness, joblessness, mental health issues, or the trauma of separation and divorce. Unfortunately it took having people that I had thought were lifelong friends desert me in my time of greatest need to realize that I myself had unwittingly passed judgement on others in my past. Paradoxically, I had people who I had been angry with for many years come to my aide. It was all beautifully confusing.

I would like to say that after I got back on my feet, I stayed there and that this book was the inspirational process on a smooth road from then on. However, just because one loses balance, falls, and gets back up, doesn't mean they won't fall again. But hopefully, they will get back up again, and again and regain the balance they lost as many times as necessary.

A year or so into my next job, my second major issue as a forty something year old physical therapist (PT) hit. Since the initial or trigger injury to my low back was at work, I also dealt with the possible stigma of being a worker's compensation patient, whom I knew from experience, certain cynical people would surmise would attempt to abuse the system. Being a PT, I felt I should have been able to avoid the injury in the first place and honestly I was embarrassed.

During past issues, I could determine for myself whether I could self diagnose and self treat or seek out the help of another therapist. This time however, I was required to go to therapy. It was very awkward to be treated by therapists in my own clinic, setting up a potential conflict of interest in my return to a full-duty workload. At the same time, if I didn't turn to them for support and chose to go to a different clinic, I felt I would be judged negatively. I had to swallow my pride on a daily basis and do the best I could in a job that was slowly beginning to have a negative rather than a positive impact on my self-esteem.

Having built my career around helping people overcome medical diagnoses that limit their mobility and function, it was quite interesting to have the table turned. I hadn't had a catastrophic life event like a stroke or a head injury. I was not suffering with a defective heart or a respiratory system, which had suffered from years of abuse. I was not afflicted with a neuromuscular disorder like Parkinson's or Cerebral Palsy. These were the problems I was used to working with and I think the most frustrating thing for me was not ever definitively getting to the root of my issues. I felt I didn't have a real problem, I just had a smattering of a bunch of different issues that added up in a big way for me. In a sense, I felt like I needed a better excuse to be struggling so much.

The possibility of MS nagged at me, knowing that often people go for years without a diagnosis and miss out on medications, which can slow down the progression of the disease. Maybe this was why I was so weak and became injured despite using good body mechanics. Possibly there was an underlying reason I was not having the strength or energy to be able to do my job the way I felt I should be able to.

However, after years of being told by significant people in my life that I was a hypochondriac, and realizing that they were probably right, I decided that if I did indeed have MS, it would eventually more obviously rear its ugly head, and in the meantime, I was going to live my life to its fullest.

Many of the fears and anxieties I had concerning my orthopedic conditions and in particular what other people may or may not have thought of me, I realize now were not healthy. What matters is being true to yourself. God knows what you're going through and what you need and as long as you trust in Him the road to healing can be much less stressful.

Actually, once I began coping with the anxiety issues of my injury as well as the physical issues, I began to heal and once again moved forward. Basically, I needed to accept I was overweight, overworked, overly stressed and over forty. Obviously there was nothing I could do to change the last condition, but certainly there were some things I could do to at least combat the former characteristics. I came across the solution to my problem during rest, relaxation, and rejuvination in my bathtub.

This book is not for a woman who dreams of being 36-24-36. Although I hope you ladies, that have attained those measurements, have done your prayers of thanksgiving, because honestly, it is just not in the genes for the majority of us. This book is for women seeking wisdom, both young and old, who just want to feel better physically and emotionally. This isn't your classic *feel-good* book. It's also a *do-good* book with a twist. For a change, you women who always are doing good for others, are going to hopefully learn to do good for yourself; and for those of us who already have enough to do, it combines the "I should do that" with an "I want to do that." Assuredly, it is tough to exercise three to four times per week. But the great majority of us hopefully bathe at least every other day.

Now you may be thinking—I don't bathe, I shower—well, there's a chapter which addresses some simple modifications to exercise in the shower. Honestly, anyways, who doesn't like a good bath every now and then? Warm bubbly water, soft lights, peace, and quiet—we really should bathe more often ladies. It is the one time that your kids will leave you alone when you're reading a good book. Of course, that is unless your children are in the toddler/preschooler-age category. Those little cuties are small enough, however, to work around in the tub if necessary. Or better yet, just play with them if they join you. There's no better exercise for both the body and the spirit than playing with your kids!

There is a disclaimer that comes with this book. Initially I was thinking I needed the disclaimer mostly for AAA personalities, but the more I got to thinking about it, I realized that I had to broaden my scope. If you are wondering what an AAA personality is, it is not people who are in desperate need for automobile assistance on a regular basis. However, I am very happy to give that particular company a plug because they have saved my butt on a multiplicity of occasions. Most of us have heard of the type A personality—the person who is ambitious, energetic, and always doing something. I have no qualms with those people, and admittedly, when I am feeling well, I am one of them. I have found myself at various points in my life, however, referring to some people (including myself if I am honest) as AAA personalities. Those are the people who push it to the limit even when it isn't good for them or anyone else, people that try and micromanage when all they need to do is trust other people a little more, and people that make the rest of us start to hyperventilate just by being around them, especially if there is a crisis or a perceived crisis at hand.

Despite the book's title, there is much information that could be helpful to men just as much as women, and although, I will typically address the females and may occasionally make a comment about our male counterpart, I believe people are people first and their gender second. That being said, women (or men) who are rule followers to the tenth degree and look at life with a very black-and-white perspective, women who are constantly trying to prove themselves, women who typically find themselves trying to rush through life to get to the next thing on their list, and women who expect miracles without having to put in the prayer time or the footwork are at risk for having difficulty absorbing some of the contents and hence benefits of this book. But it can be done, because the author of this book has at some time in her life fit into every category noted above!

Take a deep breath and know that the majority of us have struggled with at least some, if not all, of the aforementioned qualities at some point in our lives. Even if you have read plenty of self-help books and worked through such issues, it is so easy to have little relapses—let's be honest. There is hope for you to have a more peaceful and balanced life. I want this book to be about relaxing and pampering yourself, not hurting yourself. So here is the disclaimer: If any of these exercises cause discomfort or too much stress or strain, please back off! Also, most of these exercises can be done lying or sitting on your bed rather than in the tub. So if your tub is extra small, or you are extra large, no worries, enjoy reading the book in and out of the tub.

Most of the exercises that feel a bit awkward in your home tub can either be performed on dry land or a little larger water container like a Jacuzzi or a heated pool. If trying some of the exercises in a pool, sit in the corner for the exercises that use the walls of the tub for resistance, and in the very shallow end or on the steps for most of the others. There is so much more you can do aerobically in a pool than in a tub. Also, one can use water resistance when moving in a larger pool to make activities more challenging, so this book may be a little limiting in such cases, but still will provide you with many basic water exercise ideas.

Since I cannot personally meet and evaluate your issues, I will give my profession a plug here and say that if you do continue to have chronic aches and pains, it would be a good idea to ask your physician for a referral to a PT. A physical therapist can perform often-necessary soft tissue work and customize an exercise program more to your specific needs, muscular imbalances, and body type. Even if you don't experience chronic pain physically or emotionally, think of this book as a proactive approach to aging. It happens to everyone, so be prepared!

I have many times wondered in awe how my mother raised three precocious children on her own, from the time the oldest was eleven and the youngest seven. She did this on a meager secretary's salary with very little support either fiscally, physically, or emotionally from my father. We always had three square meals, clean clothes, and plenty of love. We all graduated from college with at least two different degrees and have meaningful life vocations. Mom is the proud grandma of six beautiful, bright, well-adjusted grandchildren, varying in ages from three to twenty-one years of age. She now has, among her many other accomplishments, the bittersweet accomplishment of beating cancer; not once, not twice, but three times! This is a woman with strength beyond compare.

During the writing of this book, I had an *aha* moment. I am thoroughly convinced that what got this highly organized, intense woman, who despite all her accomplishments has struggled with her self-esteem for years through her challenging life was her nightly bath-time ritual. I cannot remember a night that Mom didn't take her tub time—occasionally with teenage daughters at the mirror getting ready to head off to the movies or a football game. This was the only time I can remember Mom just relaxing, typically with a book in hand. If we couldn't come up with anything more original, we always knew bath salts or bath oil for Christmas, birthday, or Mother's Day would be much appreciated and used. And there was no giving of frivolous gifts in this family! This was a necessity!

My mom to this day is a creature of habit and discipline. I have heard it said that a successful person is a person who has good habits and I believe I agree with this statement. Ideally, the definition of success and good habits must be defined on an intrapersonal level. I tried unsuccessfully for years to create habits similar to my mom's—"early to bed, early to rise…", "cleanliness is next to Godliness", "organize your house, organize your life", etc. I am one of the most spontaneous, disorganized, yet fun-loving and creative persons I know. I am very different from my mother and it wasn't until I defined my own strengths, accepted my own weaknesses, and developed my own values, that I became successful by my own definition.

I decided one of mom's habits I could really get excited about that I had neglected through much of my life was to develop the habit of being good to myself. Seeking habits that promote balance and health in my life is what I decided to focus on. Also, I decided that daily habits can be too overwhelming for me. My mind is one that seeks novelty and variety more than consistency. Therefore, depending on the season I am in, I vary my routines.

For example, in spring and summer, there is more time devoted to gardening, biking, and walking on a regular basis and maybe a weekly bath. During the winter season, however, I decrease my outdoor activities and up my intensity of indoor exercise routines and warm relaxing baths! Another person may be a Tuesday, Thursday, Saturday bather year round. Someone else may be a binge bather—this method may come in especially handy during high-stress times. Ideally, we exercise consistently, but this book's exercise prescription is about mental health as much as it is physical and there are just times in our life when we need to practice different types of self-care. Binging on a bubble bath is much healthier than breaking out the hard alcohol or the chocolate éclairs. The secret is finding the balance that works best for you during a particular day or season of your life.

Bathing for Beginners

In the age of showering, it may be that many of you only rarely, if ever, indulge yourself with a bath. So if indeed this book inspires you to regularly recline in tub, I want to assure that you do so safely. I am a mother of three, with two in college and one not far off. My point here is, I would be delighted to make a little extra money with this project, but I do not want it to be at the cost of someone hurting themselves.

    Therefore, I am giving you all the necessary safety guidelines and implore you to use them. Accidents do happen of course, but I want to feel totally sure that they are not due to any negligence on my part. As with any exercise program, especially if you have not exercised recently or have any chronic health issues, it is recommended that you speak with a primary health care provider prior to beginning. I have based my life and career on helping, not hurting others, and my hope is that everyone who picks up this book will benefit from it in some way. As a very wise patient of mine once said, "Common sense is always in style." So let's be stylish ladies!

So, that all being said, here are a few bathtub basics:

1. If it has been years since you have gotten into a bathtub or onto the floor, may I suggest that a significant other, one of your kids or a handyman install a sturdy railing to assist with the process of getting in and out of the tub. Not to suggest that women aren't capable of home improvements, but if getting in and out of the tub is a safety hazard, chances are putting up a grab bar is too. Additionally, make sure someone is available to assist with the in-and-out process if you are unsure of your abilities.

2. Many people with balance challenges opt for sitting on a chair in the shower or bath. If you are among that group, I recommend a home consult from an exercise specialist (a physical therapist preferably) to assure the exercises in the book are modified appropriately.

3. Nonskid bath mats or bathtub stickers may safeguard against body slippage, but are not a necessity and honestly are a harbor for mold and mildew growth. If you are a person who hates cleaning the tub, I would refrain. However, I have personally found that I feel much more motivated to clean the tub when I know a nice soak can soon follow. So you need to balance for yourself the safety

of preventing a slip or preventing a UTI (urinary tract infection) that could ensue from bathing in a dirty tub. Incidentally, just to give bathing over showering another plug, per my mom, the bathing and cleaning expert, it's much easier to clean a bathed-in bath than a showered-in bath. Additionally, the bath mat or non skid stickers will interfere with the base of the tub's smooth sliding movement property utilized during a couple of exercises.

4. Keep a towel you don't mind getting wet nearby to act as a cervical (neck) or lumbar (low back) roll to make your bathing a more enjoyable and a postural correct experience. Postural correctness is the physical therapist's version of political correctness. If you are not doing exercises with proper posture, some therapists will say you might as well not be exercising at all. So there will be a brief tutorial on bathtub posture following. The towel will come in handy for a couple of different exercises as well.

5. Candles, a glass of wine or your favorite beverage, and sweet-smelling bubble bath, bath fizz, or shower gel (whatever your toiletry of choice) is not a requirement, but highly recommended. It is easier to get dehydrated when your body is submersed in water so be sure to either drink plenty of nonalcoholic and non-caffeinated beverages prior, during, and/or after any exercise. Crisp clear water is

always your best option—the spout is within arms reach!

6. When I am referring to different areas of the tub while explaining exercises, keep the following basic definitions in mind. Pretty basic, but I just want to clarify:

   A. Front wall of tub—where the water spigot comes out
   B. Back wall of tub—opposite above, usually an angled wall
   C. Side walls of tub—right and left
   D. Back/front/side wall edges—horizontal part

Now for my tutorial on Postural Correctness: I recommend you practice as you read.

Upright Sitting: In this position, your hips should be closer to the back of the tub. Your spine should be erect and not resting on the back wall of the tub with the possible exception of your sacrum (essentially the base of your spine and the back of your pelvis/hips). Your shoulder blades should be down and back, to avoid a slouched upper trunk. Think of pulling your should blades down toward your buttocks. And finally, your chin should be tucked. To do a proper chin tuck, look straight ahead while gently pulling your head back without looking up, as if you are gently holding an orange/apple/egg under your chin. If you have poor posture at baseline this may feel quite awkward to you; but with time and continuing to strengthen weak muscles it will feel more natural.

Reclined: In this position, allow your hips to slide toward the center of the tub and rest your spine on the back wall of the tub. Unless you have a very biomechanically correct tub (which I have yet to discover) to virtually allow you to be in long sitting with your back fully supported and your neck resting on the back edge of the tub, this could be a problematic position for your neck and low back. So if you have any tendency towards issues in either or both of these areas, you may need a rolled towel placed in the curve behind your neck and or your low back for extra support. Typically, however, the buoyancy of the water is sufficient, unless you're a sinker.

One last detail before we get to work. I have some recommendations as to how to utilize this book. Initially, I would like you to read through the book one to three chapters at a time in a leisurely fashion in whatever time permits for you. Remember, this book is about being good to yourself and getting to know your body. It is not about seeing how much you can do in as short a time possible. You need to learn how to just relax and get comfortable in the tub with good posture. Enjoy my ramblings as food for your mind as you intersperse some exercises to alert your body, and take in what you are meant to learn. Take moments to just close your eyes and be quiet within yourself as the mood moves you.

After you get through the book once, at the end, there is a sequential guide to getting through an entire bath-time workout in about twenty to thirty minutes. There are page references to get more specific instructions on each exercise. Please do not rush to the back of the book and flip forward for reference without reading through the entire book first, as you may miss important points for your health and safety.

So let's now begin with our first exercise! Now, don't get too excited, as we're going to start slow. Our first exercise is about breathing. You will use this exercise virtually with every other exercise that follows. Now, I am not trying to insult your intelligence here. True, if you weren't breathing already, you obviously would not be able to read this book. However, you would be shocked by how many people actually breathe incorrectly without even utilizing their strongest breathing muscle, the diaphragm. Other times, people actually hold their breath during muscular contractions, which can be quite hard on the heart, especially if the exercise is a stressful one. One of the most common things I have to say to my patients, especially after surgery, when a muscular contraction may be quite painful is "Breathe!"

Deep breathing is the key to relaxation or coping when you are stressed, sad, angry, nervous, bored, frustrated, exhausted, confused, embarrassed, frightened, overwhelmed, anxious, or even hysterical. Whether these emotions are instigated by a positive or negative event, breathing is essential to getting yourself to a state where you can think clearly and act calmly. Ironically, some people do not even realize they are feeling such sentiments until they find themselves taking a deep cleansing breath or notice that their neck and shoulders are feeling particularly sensitive or painful as we tend to tense up when we feel strong emotions.

The primary muscles used in breathing are the diaphragm and also the intercostal (translates to *between ribs*) muscles. Many people additionally use accessory breathing muscles if they are stressed, respiratory wise due to illness, exertion, or just plain bad habits. A commonly used accessory muscle to avoid activating during deep breathing is the trapezius (shortened commonly to *traps*). These are the muscles that elevate your shoulders, as in a shrug. Chances are if you are utilizing your traps to take a deep breath, you aren't using your diaphragm, which is our most efficient respiratory muscle. If you find yourself pulling your shoulders up toward your ears when you breathe deeply, it may be helpful to precede your deep breathing exercises with shoulder rolls to get your traps to relax.

For the next few exercises, I want you to be in the most relaxed and aligned position of your preference, either in upright sitting or reclined, paying attention to postural correctness. Or you may choose to be more buoyant with your upper body, floating in the water and your legs flexed (bent) and relaxed.

- *Shoulder Rolls*: Simply roll your shoulders backward and pinch your shoulder blades together. Be sure that your chin is tucked while you do your shoulder rolls. Repeat multiple times synchronizing shoulder rolls with slow, gentle breathing through your mouth or nose and repeat until you feel relaxed. You can also roll your shoulders forward, but I personally find this awkward. The forward roll actually feeds into the incorrect forward shoulder posture which is problematic for many, especially as one ages and begins the fight against gravity. The pectoral muscle, fondly referred to as "pecs," is typically too tight in the majority of individuals so backward rolls are the priority.
- *Diaphragmatic/Deep Breathing*: The diaphragm is one of the few muscles in the body, which originates from bone, but does not insert onto bone. The diaphragm is shaped like a conical donut, with the center being a ring of connective tissue surrounding the major abdominal vessels through which oxygenated and deoxygenated blood passes.
  1. As a person inhales and the lungs fill with air, the diaphragm flattens, thus pushing downward on your stomach and intestines and pooching out your abdomen. As you exhale, if you are utilizing your diaphragm to take that deep breath, your belly should flatten slightly.

2. People that are shallow breathers tend to breathe in and out through their mouths. A cue to remember in order to take an efficient deep breath is to breathe in through your nose as if smelling the roses, chocolate chip cookies, an ocean breeze—whatever tickles your fancy—and then a long steady breath out through your mouth like you're blowing out birthday candles or bubbles. Try to envision the sight and the smell of something positive and calming to you. When you exercise, attempt to get your breathing in sync with repetitions of the exercises to assure good blood flow to your muscles and through your cardiorespiratory system.

3. To simplify, in through the nose with a slow count of three, out through the mouth with a slow count of six. Repeat.

- *Neck Range of Motion:* This is a personal favorite of mine due to my history of neck issues. If you are not in a buoyant position already, slide your hips toward the center of the tub. Depending on your height, you may choose to rest your legs on the front edge or walls of the tub, or let your legs rest in a *crisscross applesauce* position (kindergarten flashback)—whatever is most comfortable. The idea is to get your head totally relaxed and buoyant in the water.

1. Now gently turn your head as far to the left and then the right as possible, being careful to keep your nose either above water or exhaling during underwater activities (grade school flashback). Repeat several times, attempting to turn your head a little farther each time, especially if your nose is far from reaching the water's edge, which would indicate that you have limited range of motion in your cervical spine.

2. I also enjoy extending my neck as far as possible in this position. Many of us are frequently looking down throughout the day and rarely look up. This can be very stressful to your cervical disks incidentally. You may want to stabilize yourself with your elbows on the base of the tub. Then stretch your neck backwards, taking note of any mold or mildew on the ceiling, which you (or preferably a teenager who is being punished) may want to scrub off later.

3. Next, with your head still buoyant, cock your neck side to side, directing your ear to the right then left shoulder.

4. In summary, turn neck, extend neck, cock neck, repeating ten to thirty times each.

Incidentally, especially if you have issues with neck pain or arthritis, you may find that attempting to do these neck range of motion exercises out of water is a bit more stressful than in water. Water's gravity eliminating properties can assist you in maintaining pain free range of motion. However, by doing these exercises in the water, the joint grinding/clunking sounds which are the hallmark of arthritis may be audible. If that bothers you, which it does me, just perform the range of motion exercises slower and the sound shouldn't be as dramatic. It is even more important to do this particular group of exercises if you are hearing such joint crepitus in your neck. If you are having a day with a particularly stiff neck, try looping a towel around you neck and hold either end of the towel with your hands to give your neck a little extra support while you do your range exercises.

When life gets tough, as it unfortunately sometimes will, no matter where you are—the bathtub, the backyard, the boss's office—you can always breathe deeply to bring yourself back to that inner peaceful place. If you practice these breathing techniques and relaxation exercises on a regular basis, they will become more automatic and ward off the turmoil and chaos that can plague your spirit.

One thing I have learned in the fourth and fifth decades of my life is that the notion I had as a teenager that life would get easier the older I got, was not necessarily true. I finally understand that this thing we call life is typically quite complicated. But if we meet each day sincerely doing the best we can to be good to both ourselves and others we will eventually begin feeling at peace. Contentment with whatever the day brings will be ours. God will give us the strength and the tools to deal with whatever comes along. We just need to pay attention to his prodding and breathe deeply when we feel confused and alone. There we will find him in the midst of it all.

Stretch Yourself

Stretch yourself–push the limits–be flexible–move out of your comfort zone; these phrases are all synonymous with putting oneself through a bit of discomfort–be it mentally, physically, or emotionally– in order to reach a better place. Stretching your muscles to become more flexible as well requires a bit of discomfort.

Now, for those of you who dislike pain, which covers the great majority of us, I must do a little instruction here on one of healthcare's favorite tools—the pain scale. It entails ranking pain on a scale from zero to ten, with zero being no pain and ten being the most excruciating pain one can imagine. This tool can be very helpful for diagnosing and treatment, if used accurately. However, that can be a challenge.

I must admit it is a pet peeve of mine when I ask a patient to rank their pain on the scale and I get the answer ten, with a smile no less. Agh! You could not smile let alone even speak if your pain was a ten on the pain scale. Sometimes people are just being over dramatic or attempting to interject humor into their unhappy situation. Sometimes there is a patient who simply has difficulty processing such gray zones or they may be a bit foggy and confused (quite common after surgery). Most likely however, someone may not be understanding the importance of ranking pain accurately and being in tune with the mind-body connection.

Unfortunately the scream of, *"My pain is at a ten– do something!"* is often seen as a red flag rather than a physical emergency. The medical profession needs to be constantly vigilant for *drug seeking behavior* of people addicted to medications. This problem has sadly reached epidemic proportions in today's society and can result in loss of life. Ironically, the healthcare industry is largely to blame for its own crisis due to overmedicating and over prescribing highly addictive narcotics. There are many alternative pain medications other than narcotics, as well as methods to deal with pain that do not involve medications.

Pain is an extremely complicated concept. There are physiological and psychological issues that impact both pain levels and a person's ability to cope with pain. Pain has an important purpose to alert us to danger. However, it is very common for a person to become over focused on their pain, and hence create more anxiety and more pain that is no longer productive pain. Productive pain serves the purpose of alerting us to a problem. Regrettably, pain can easily and unnecessarily transition from productive pain to pain that is only limiting us physically and emotionally. I have experienced both types of pain and realize that at times it is very difficult to discern which is going on. The relaxation techniques such as shoulder rolls and deep breathing described in the previous chapter can often dampen physical pain that is being worsened psychologically. In any case, it is important to have pain evaluated by your doctor to determine if further assessment is needed.

Surprisingly, there is such a thing as good pain. Level one to three pain (dependent on your personal pain tolerance) on the zero to ten scale that occurs during stretching is an indicator that you are doing a stretch correctly. The burn you get during aerobic activity or strengthening is also a good pain and a sign that you are building muscle tissue. If during stretching, your pain creeps above a three, that's a sign to back off, however. Additionally, if during or after exercise your pain creeps above a three and does not calm down after about twenty minutes of rest, that is an indicator that you have potentially injured yourself or overdone it. But during a stretch you should feel something, or you likely are not doing the exercise correctly.

Depending on where your muscle tightness is, stretches may elicit a mild pull or pain in different areas. Occasionally, if you are adequately flexible or overstretched in a certain muscle group, you may not feel a stretch or you may feel a strain somewhere other than where it is indicated. Likely however, if you don't feel the stretch, it is because your postural alignment is lacking. So if you don't feel the pull, try straightening your spine, aligning your pelvis, or straightening your knee, whichever gets the indicated outcome.

For those of us ladies that are habitual multitaskers and like to use our time efficiently, you should appreciate the following two exercises which may be done in conjunction with shaving your legs (hamstring stretch) or shaving your armpits (triceps stretch). Conveniently, the time it takes to fully shave your lower extremity is a good duration for a static stretch—thirty seconds to one minute. Before we move on to the exercise explanation however, I have a comment or two on multitasking.

In my opinion, multitasking, like any other skill, has different levels of proficiency. Some of us are gifted at this task, and others, well not so much. Men in particular are typically quite challenged in this area, being about as good at multitasking as they are at accessorizing. No insult intended here. To a man's credit, they may not multitask as often as we females, and that is often a good thing. Especially in this case, as I think most of us women would agree that although we may like clean-shaven men, this would be taking things a little too far.

Warning to the women though—it is quite difficult to keep in balance while simultaneously performing three different tasks at once. It is wise to not attempt multitasking until you have proficiency in the skills separately and totally fine to do these stretches in isolation. I do not want us feeling like teenage girls again with multiple razor wounds in sensitive areas.

Triceps Stretch:

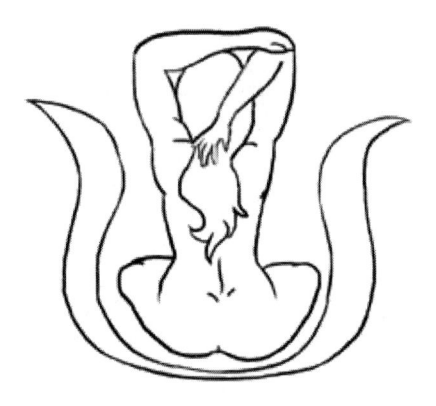

- Assume the typical armpit-shaving position.

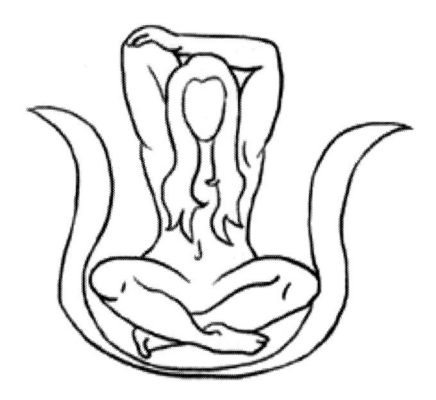

- Instead of just holding your arm straight up, bend at your elbow so that your hand drops behind your shoulder blade.

- Push back on your elbow with the opposite hand. If you choose to continue holding the razor during this seemingly simple upper-extremity-coordination activity, beware of sharp razor blades.
- Repeat with opposite extremity.
- Hold stretch for thirty seconds to one minute.

Hamstring Stretch:

- Assume the typical leg shaving position.
- Instead of bending your knee, keep your knee straight, tightening your knee cap.
- Raise your leg straight up so you feel a pull behind your knee and thigh. You can be reclined and pull the leg up straight above you. Or you can be in a upright sitting position with your heel resting on the ledge of the tub. Remember to bend primarily at the the hips, keeping your spine and knee as straight as possible.
- Then shave away while holding the stretch for thirty seconds to one minute!
- To reach the sides of your legs, rather than bending at the knee, you can rotate at your hip and/ or cross your leg over the midline of your body for a little additional hip stretch.

The following positional stretches are simply different sitting positions that can usually be done in the bathtub, depending on its size and your proportions, but also can be performed sitting on the floor or in bed with good pelvic posture. Proper pelvic posture entails being sure you are actually sitting on the bones that you were designed by our good Lord to sit on. If you sit up straight and poke yourself in the center of your bum, you will feel your ischial tuberosities (pronounced ish-ee-ul tubes for short).

Many people sit on their tailbone (coccyx) or their sacrum when they are slouching. These two areas are the most common place that our thin-skinned deconditioned geriatric population gets bedsores, or *sloppy sitting sores*. Now is the time to ingrain good pelvic posture into your muscle memory, as the older we get, the less muscle elasticity we have, and the more difficulty we will have in altering our poor body mechanics and posture. The sitting positions below are wonderful stretches in and of themselves as long as you are paying attention to your *pelvic posture*. Remember, as you're sitting, sit on your *ischial tubes*.

Sole Sitting:

This may initially be a difficult position with a narrow bathtub unless you have very good hip range of motion or are quite petite. Proceed gradually with this exercise as explained below to determine if you have the range of motion to sit safely in this position. Additionally, it is important to keep an erect spine to gain the full benefit of this stretch.

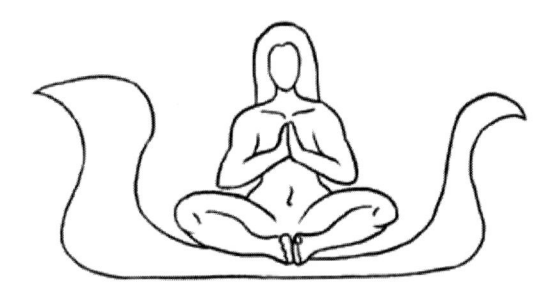

- Begin by sitting diagonally in the tub with your shins crossed over another.
- Your goal is to eventually get yourself turned sideways in the tub with the soles of your feet touching, as in the above picture, but you may have to wait a few weeks to gain enough flexibility to tolerate the soles touching position.
- The first transition will be to get yourself sitting sideways rather than diagonally, facing out of the tub with your legs crossed at your ankles.
- During this transition, place both your hands behind you on the floor of the tub so that you can more easily shift your weight.
- Straighten your elbows and lift left hip off the base of the tub so you can shift your weight to the right hip and pull your legs further apart. Do this weight shift incrementally

- while simultaneously turning your body to face out of the tub.

- Once you get one ankle on top of the other comfortably, you are ready to move to the point that your soles are touching and the side of the bathtub is helping you stretch your inner thighs fully.

- Again place your hands behind your buttocks and straighten your elbows. Now pull your knees further apart and join the soles of your feet, keeping your toes splayed rather than curled to avoid a cramp in the arch of your foot.

- If the soles-touching position is too much for you, just sit in an intermediary positions working on gradually bringing your feet closer together and knees wider apart. With practice, the transition into sole sitting will become easier.

- Once in a comfortable position feeling a gentle stretch, focus on good spinal posture. Then place your hands either centrally or relaxed on your knees and thighs and breathe deeply for about ten repetitions.

- Eventually when you reach the soles touching position, you can push your knees down toward the floor of the tub to increase the stretch.

Side Sitting:

Side sitting is my personal favorite. Even on days when I have already done a full workout in a different venue, or simply feel I am out of balance and need relaxation more than exercise, I often will hold this position for a few minutes stretch before ending my bath-time ritual. I like to totally rest my body in this position by placing both my forearms up on the front or back ledge of the tub and rest my forehead on my arms. This is a great trunk rotation stretch and a good position to work on deep breathing.

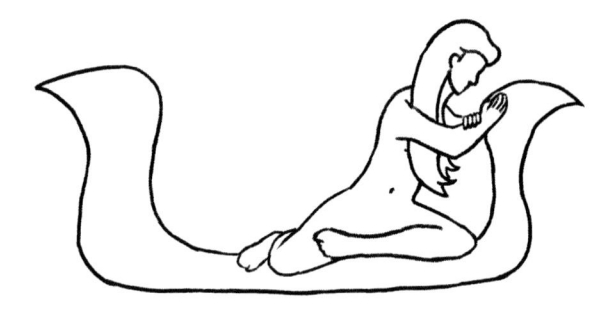

- Begin by sitting long ways in the tub and bending both knees.
- While turning to face out of the tub, let both knees drop to one side so that you are sitting on one hip.
- Separate your legs in this side sitting position so that your foot is just below the knee or slightly in front of the thigh of the opposite

leg. The closer your foot is toward your groin, the more stretch you will get to your hip.

- For some of you, this may be enough stretch in and of itself and you may find yourself placing your hand down on the base of the tub to prop yourself up if you have weak or fatigued abdominals.
- If a further stretch is desired, place one forearm on the back ledge of the tub and your other hand on the floor of the tub. Both forearms on the back ledge is also an option.
- Then you can rest your forehead on your forearm(s) and breathe deeply.
- Repeat stretch in above sequence, dropping legs to opposite side.

Long Sitting:

1. Sit up nice and tall.
2. Straighten your legs out in front of you, keeping the backs of your knees on the base of the tub.
3. Draw your toes up toward your shins while keeping your knees straight and reach toward your toes.

It's as simple as one, two, three! As you do this stretch regularly you will find yourself being able to reach further down your shins to your ankles, instep, then toes without your knees wanting to bend.

Piriformis Stretch:

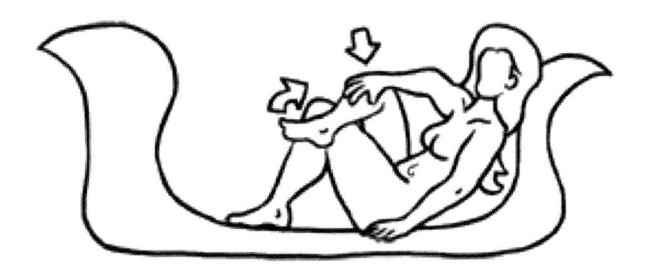

Another stretch we are going to cover is an important one for people who have recurrent *sciatica*. Sciatica is a general term used to describe pain that radiates down a leg, usually originating from a back or hip problem. The piriformis is often the muscle that is the culprit for causing such problems. The sciatic nerve passes through the center of this small triangular muscle. If this muscle is tight, it is more prone to have spasms, especially if you have any spine problems. So keeping it flexible can help to prevent or combat such difficulties. The side sitting stretch can also stretch this muscle once spinal muscles are sufficiently flexible.

- Begin in a reclined position with your right knee bent and the right foot flat on the floor of the tub.
- Place your left outer ankle on top of the right thigh.
- Lift the right foot off the base of the tub, and push/pull your legs up toward your chest.

- Your left leg should fall to the side. Place your hand on your left knee to cue yourself.
- You should feel a good stretch in your left buttocks.
- Hold for 30-60 seconds then repeat with your left foot on the base of the tub and right ankle resting on left thigh.

Shoulder Extension Stretch:

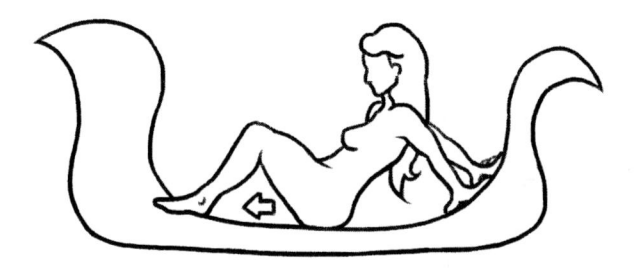

Unless you are an avid ball player or swimmer, the likelihood is you don't often extend either of your shoulders to their maximum potential. Tight shoulders often lead to hunched shoulders, which often leads to poor upper back posture. This stretch may be difficult for some people to do initially, in which case, rather than placing your hands on the ledge of the bathtub, place them on the floor of the bathtub in the corners.

- Begin by sitting upright in the center of the tub.

- Reach back, one hand at a time toward the back of the tub with your palms facing down. (For more of a stretch, rest your hands on the ledge of the tub, for less stretch on the base of the tub.)
- Straighten your elbows and slide your hips toward your feet as much as possible so that you feel a gentle pull in the front of your shoulders.
- Hold for thirty to sixty 30-60 seconds, then release one hand at a time.
- For the most benefit, keep your trunk and neck erect/extended.

More dynamic stretches will be incorporated throughout the rest of the book, but these few should get you started. Flexibility is not only important to our physical bodies, but also for our life to be fulfilling. Being a rigid person rarely helps you to experience all life has to offer. Spontaneity and willingness to compromise keeps a multiplicity of options open in life.

There is so much to experience and the more flexible you are the more opportunities you likely will have. However, it is important to have both strength and flexibility, to stay in balance and for your life and body to run relatively smoothly and injury-free. One must learn to discern that certain times call for strength and standing your ground while other times call for flexibility and moving from your initial position. This is a skill which can be developed through prayer and self control. Pausing to breathe deeply and ask to be filled with the Holy Spirit before deciding which is the wisest course of action comes with time and practice.

The next few chapters will focus on strengthening various body parts. The order of the chapters or your workout is not necessarily important, but be sure not to neglect a certain body part. Every bit of you is important!

Upper Body Urgency

Hate to tell you this ladies, but we're not getting any younger. It's important to start dealing with the inevitable. If you are in my target audience of middle-aged mamas, then grandmahood is just around the corner. And believe me, it can be a scary sight. I am talking serious regression here. Remember those cute little diapers we used to put on our babies? And how about those toddler walkers with all the little spinning toys our kids used to push around? These concepts, although often necessary, are not so cute in the over seventy population.

That being said, I have seen many women over seventy, my own mother included, in better shape than me, so there is a hope! An old friend of mine liked to bring up the fact that we, humans, are the only species in which the female continues to be a productive member of the pack long after childbearing years have passed. Following menopause, most female mammals die off soon after, but not us Homo sapiens. We not only stay alive, but we can thrive! This time of life is an opportunity for women to redefine themselves.

Even if we are among the *working-out-of-the-home* moms group, during our children's childhood and adolescence, our priority is typically our kids, and career comes second. Now your priority can be yourself! If motherhood has not been a part of your life to this point, menopause might be even more difficult. Whether the decision to not be a mother was yours, or not, often one may find themselves asking questions about where her life journey has taken her and where it is going during this next phase.

I personally was one of those working moms who felt guilty not being a stay-at-home mom. I ran myself ragged trying to do everything, and sometimes more, to make up for the fact that I wasn't one of those mom's who we saw on TV with cookies, a spotless house, and a fun project or outing, awaiting the kids when they jumped off the school bus. Then there is the other end of the spectrum— the stay-at-home mom that feels inadequate because she never got her college degree or *did anything* with it. Every Mom is a working mom, and it is hard work! I believe being a Mom is the toughest, most rewarding and most important job all rolled into one that a woman can have. Personally, I believe raising well-rounded, well-balanced, and well-adjusted children, or being such a person yourself, is the biggest feat any woman can accomplish. And when that responsibility is completed or near completion, many women find themselves struggling with their identity and their purpose.

Middle age can be even more difficult if your young adult children are struggling a bit with their own life purpose and direction and making choices you find a bit disturbing. Know that you did the best you could with the resources you had at the time and take comfort in the fact that you are not alone. Even the so-called perfect parent can have a child who struggles. More importantly, take comfort in knowing that God isn't done with them yet. Take comfort in knowing that even if your beautiful baby, all grown up, no longer wants to be a part of your life, just so long as you can forgive them for that and continue to lift them up in prayer, God will keep his promises to you. Have faith in His ability to set your son or daughter back on the right path once they have learned the lessons that they need to learn. We as parents cannot always teach them everything. While they are away learning about life, you can continue to do the same and when reconciliation comes, you will have all the more love to share.

Time spent in the bathtub, between reading and exercising of course, is a great opportunity to dream and plan where your life goes from here—whether you're twenty-three or seventy-three, or somewhere in between. None of us know how long this gift of life will be ours to share. None of us know what tomorrow has in store. In my opinion, the secret to a happy life is having no regrets about the past, acknowledging mistakes and learning from them, living in the moment, and alleviating anxiety about the future by anticipating tomorrow with joyful hope.

This is the time to make a plug about developing your own personal life motto. Mine is "Patience and Persistence Balanced in Love." At one point, I had a little teeter-totter with a capital *P* on either side, and a heart for a fulcrum taped on my bathroom mirror just to remind me. Earlier in the book, I had a little picture of my balance scale with two Ps and a triangle. Whether a triangle or a heart, it can pretty much represent the same thing as I think about a triangle representing The Trinity, which I believe represents Love.

PP_____PP
▲

I have since added a couple other Ps to my scale. Positive Attitude and Peacefulness are my current focuses. Although I continue to have a need to practice patience and persistence in my slightly zany life with two adult children living in our home, one of whom brought a fourth dog to add to our pack when she returned. When I first returned to my home of origin, it became abundantly clear that I needed to make a couple additions to my motto as the reconciliation wasn't as smooth as I would have liked it to be. Believe me it took more than just the four Ps. It really was the base of the scale that was the biggest factor in keeping my peace.

My priest recently described the mystery of the Trinity, the Father, the Son, and the Holy Spirit as "three persons bound in a relationship of love." He went on to explain that we, as Christians, can reflect God's image in our own lives, even if it is just a brief glimpse in comparison. The mystery of God's profound Love, through the Holy Trinity only gets deeper and more expansive as we reflect on it and continue sharing the infinite love he has given us to spread during our finite lives. If all relationships could be based on the idea of a trinitarian love, how much easier relationships could be.

My little life motto is now such an integral part of who I strive to be that I no longer need a visual aid. At one point, however, when my depression and anxiety was a constant battle within me, that little motto helped me to face days and nights that I didn't want to face. It helped me to get myself out of bed after an insomniatic night of one or two hours sleep. It helped me to not let myself overdose on the medication that was suppose to make me better. It helped me to put one foot in front of the other and get out the door to a job where I had to cope with the suffering of others which in comparison to mine was often much greater but which also made my emotional lability much worse. My simple life motto helped me to wipe away my tears and try to look toward each new day with hope.

If determining a life motto seems too daunting, may I suggest making a *Bathtub Bucket List*. Writing a book has always been on my personal bucket list and I'm sure it's not surprising that the inspiration for this book came during one of my personal training sessions in the tub. Hopefully the publishing of this book just might lead to checking other things off my bucket list and I hope reading this book will inspire many of you to tackle your bucket list as well.

So to get back to the topic—the reason I titled this chapter "Upper Body Urgency": It is a physiological fact that we women will rarely compare to our male counterparts when it comes to upper body strength. That does not mean to imply that upper body strength is not important. Just because something doesn't come naturally to us, this does not mean it is not an important area in our overall health and well-being. Upper body strength is very important.

If you have a history of neck problems, the likelihood is that you have weak arms and do a lot of substitution with a very large muscle called the *trapezius*. This is that muscle that we "Ooh and aah" about when someone comes up behind us and puts their hands on either side of our neck and gives us a quick rub. You know who you are—it hurts so good type of feeling—you my dears likely have weak biceps, triceps, external rotators (I'll explain that more later) and over use your traps. So they are tired and overworked, which leads to muscle tension and poor posture and that "Oh, my neck," which is of course attached to the "Oh, my aching back" frequent phrase. I have been one of those women. Despite being a very well-trained PT, I did not specialize in orthopedics. I specialized in neurology essentially, and although these two systems do not work in isolation, I was neglectful of taking care of my upper body balance.

Working back in geriatrics again for a few years after a long stint in pediatrics was quite the eye opener for me. I had lost my perspective not being around our sweet little old ladies who in their eighties are four feet ten inches although they swear at one point they were five feet five inches. When vertebrae begin collapsing and hunched posture ensues, it not only affects one's height, but it also affects the ability to take a nice deep breath, the ability of one's stomach and intestines to empty easily and a host of other problems.

Collapsing vertebrae is not only due to years and years of muscular imbalances, but osteoporosis setting in. Some osteoporosis is due to genetics, some calcium intake as a child and an adult, and some how much weight-bearing activity you have had over the years. Additionally, let us not forget those wonderful female hormone fluctuations we experience throughout our lives and then the resultant depletion of them. So each of us ladies will eventually have at least one of these four major risk factors.

Every single one of us has about a ten percent chance of breaking a hip if we live over the age of eighty. Now these are pretty daunting odds. We should do all we can now to avoid being in that ten percent statistic. Reading this book and following its recommendations may help to decrease those odds. Unfortunately, however, even the most-prepared individual can get caught in a bad storm. So if you're a future hip casualty, having a strong upper body will definitely help you through the rehab process and decrease the high morbidity rate that accompanies a hip fracture.

Dependent on the type of fracture one has, the orthopedist will either cut off the top of the femur (thigh bone), taking off the ball portion of the ball-and-socket joint, essentially replacing the hip joint, or he will put a customized selection of screws, nails, plates, and rods inside to hold things together. Either way, going through airport security will never be the same. Either way, there will be a lot of pain (unless one has a particularly superb surgeon and a particularly high pain tolerance). Either way, a walker or crutches will be needed for at least two months if not the rest of life. And either way, you will need strong arms to compensate for the fact that for at least a while, your leg is not going to be able to take the full weight of your body. Just a side note, if the surgeon were to give an option to decide between a new joint or nails and pins, (whether that would be an option would depend on the type of fracture), I would recommend opting for the new joint as the rehab process tends to be much easier.

Speaking of a new joint, if you are one of the lucky ones to make it into your eighties without a hip fracture, there is the high likelihood that you will have some amount of arthritis. The majority of the exercises in this book are very conducive to that diagnosis. Hopefully, exercising appropriately on a regular basis can help to prevent such drastic measures as a total hip, total knee, total shoulder, or spinal fusion that many individuals with arthritis eventually resort to.

It is an interesting observation that one can look at two different sets of x-rays, one with what looks like it should be debilitating arthritis and another that has mild-to-moderate arthritis, and the person with the more severe arthritis may report less pain and more function than the person with more mild bone and cartilage changes. This has a lot to do with the health of the tissues surrounding that joint and the health of the blood and nerve supply feeding that joint and the muscles, tendons and ligaments that surround it. And the health of all those systems has a lot to do with having a regular exercise program.

Sometimes, despite what you do, it may be inevitable that you will have to eventually go *under the knife*. But then again, the outcome of that procedure will have a lot to do with not only how well you follow the rehabilitation recommendations, but also how healthy your muscles and other tissues were prior to the operation. Another side note here, if you are planning to have or recently had surgery, check with your personal physician and/or physical therapist about the appropriateness or modifications of some of the exercises in this book for your specific needs.

So let us proceed to the upper body exercises. If there is more than one exercise for a certain muscle group, the easier exercise will be listed first, which will typically be of the isometric form. There is a threefold reason for the frequency of isometric exercises in this book: ease of learning, therapeutic benefit, and the convenience of the bathtub walls in facilitating this type of exercise. Iso means *the same*, metric means *distance*. So an isometric exercise means that the muscle fibers are not shortening or lengthening, they are contracting, but not changing significantly in shape. Basically, by using the resistance of the bathtub wall you can get a good muscle contraction without moving your joint significantly. This is an excellent form of strengthening for people with arthritic and/or painful joints. However, if you are in a hot tub or a pool and have more space to move through a full arc of motion, moving quickly can offer some resistance from the water without unduly stressing the joint. Therefore I will feature both isometric and other exercises that offer more range of motion for each muscle group as it is appropriate.

The first muscle group we will address is the elbow flexors, commonly referred to as the *biceps*. However there are half a dozen different muscles that assist in bending your elbow. The biceps gets the most credit because it is the bulkiest, but bulk doesn't necessarily translate to best. Actually, the biceps tendon muscle is known to rupture, leaving the muscle basically useless and typically there is no surgical intervention as the other muscles substitute quite well.

Since this muscle group is quite strong, you will need some bathtub props to assist in sufficient strengthening. You have two convenient options—shampoo and conditioner bottles and towels. Bottles of varying amounts of content make great weights for the following exercises. If you are having to do greater than twenty repetitions to begin to feel like you are expending any effort, then a wet towel is an additional option. The trick to getting the most out of these exercises is to move slowly with control.

Bicep Curls

This exercise can be done with right and left arm simultaneously, alternating right and left, or isolating one arm at a time.

- Begin in an upright sitting position
- Tuck your elbow(s) at your side.
- With hands fisted or holding weights, bend your elbow(s) fully and hold tightly for a count of three to five seconds.
- Slowly lower hands to base of tub
- Rest and repeat until fatigued, likely 10-30 repetitions.

Shampoo Shuffle:

Most bathtubs have that shelf that is just out of reach and that was the inspiration for this exercise as I had to do a total body weight shift in order to reach the desired beauty product and found myself doing not only a good arm exercise, but exercising my trunk as well. Care should be taken as over-reaching can be dangerous to the shoulder complex so assure that you move slowly and don't push into discomfort.

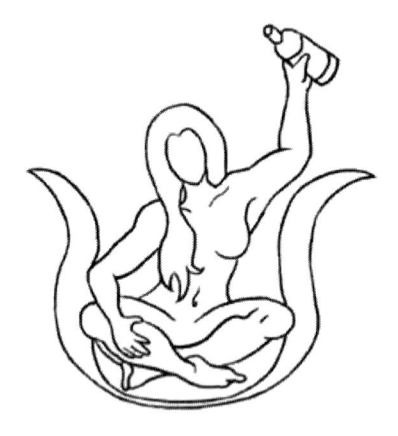

- Begin in an upright sitting position with knees relaxed.
- Shift your weight onto your right hip and reach high over your head with your right arm so that the right side of your trunk is elongating and the left side of your trunk is shortening.
- Lower your right arm and if you choose to use shampoo bottles as weights, transfer the bottle from your right hand to your left hand.
- Shift weight to left hip and reach up then lower left arm, lengthening the left trunk and shortening on the right.
- Repeat, alternating sides for 10-30 repetitions.
- This exercise can also be done in the kneeling position. While reaching up come into a tall kneeling position and when lowering your

arm move into low kneeling so your bum is resting on your heels.

If you are of the opinion that less is more or you have a day in which you are unable to do your full workout, I would prioritize the triceps ahead of the biceps in the importance of upper body exercises. These are the most important *crutch gait* muscles that hopefully you will never have to rely on for weight-bearing activities with crutches or a walker. Additionally, they are in the area of *flabby underarm syndrome* that many women complain about, so toning up your triceps has dual benefit. The next three exercises all strengthen the triceps. They are listed in order of difficulty, with the easiest being the isometric triceps and the most difficult being the reverse push-ups.

Isometric Triceps:

- Assume an upright sitting posture with your palms on the base of the tub behind your buttocks or:
- Assume a reclined sitting position with your hands next to your thighs.
- Push your hands into the base of the tub so that you feel a tightening in the back of your upper arms.
- You may straighten your elbows but try not to hitch your shoulders up toward your ears.

- Hold for a 3-5 count and repeat until muscle begins to feel fatigued, likely 10-30 repetitions.

Antigravity Triceps:

You may want to use weights for this exercise as in the biceps curl. Antigravity triceps can be done alternating right and left, simultaneously, or in isolation.

- Raise your arm so your forearm is next to the ear and your elbow is bent so your hand is behind your shoulder.
- Straighten the elbow fully to raise your hand above the head while turning your palm so it is facing upward.
- Lower elbow to a bent position slowly and repeat 10-30x.

Reverse push-ups

This exercise is a progression basically of the isometric triceps.

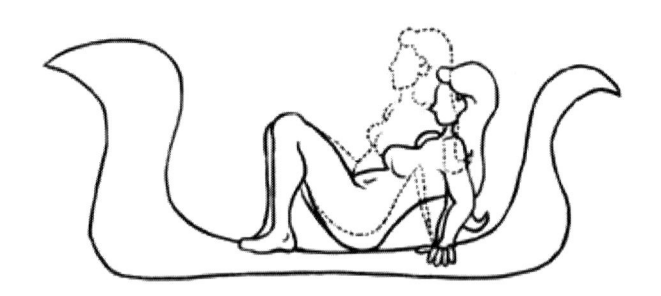

- Begin in an upright sitting posture with your palms on the base of the tub behind your buttocks. You may want to recline back slightly.
- Fully straighten your elbow.
- Instead of allowing your shoulders to hike up toward your ears, keep your shoulders down and raise your bum off the base of the tub.
- Repeat 10–30x

The shoulder is one of the most complex and mobile joints in our body. It also is not just one joint. Most of our joints are the articulation of two different bones on one another. The movement of the shoulder actually has multiple bones involved: the collarbone(clavicle), the shoulder blade(scapula), the breast bone(sternum) and the upper rib cage all act in concert with the humerus (upper arm bone). There are also a multiplicity of muscles involved in the movement of the shoulder girdle. The single biggest culprit for shoulder problems are weak external rotators. These are the small muscles that in part make up the rotator cuff. Often they are not as strong as they should be, hence the greater likelihood that those muscles can tear or that impingement syndromes can occur because of faulty biomechanics. I have treated extremely muscular young men (typically football players) who look very strong, but have very weak external rotators of their shoulder girdle. Following is a very simple, yet a very important exercise that should be done on a regular basis to prevent shoulder problems.

Isometric External Rotators

- Assume an upright sitting or semi-reclined position.
- Let your forearms rest on your stomach, then while keeping elbows tucked, move your forearms toward the sidewalls of the tub, rotating at your shoulders, keeping your thumbs pointing up.
- Keep your elbows tucked at your side.
- Push into the sidewalls of the tub with the same rotational movement.
- Hold for a count of 3-5 then rest and repeat 10-30x.

Now that we've worked the external rotators, I have a simple exercise to work their counterparts, the internal rotators. This does not need to be done in the bathtub necessarily. I would actually just recommend doing it at least once a day or whenever you feel the need. We've all heard the phrase "Have you hugged your kids today?" Well how about "Have you hugged yourself today?" I recently heard on my favorite radio station—KLOVE (It's a national station and online—look it up if you're not familiar)—that hugging yourself once a day significantly reduces stress hormones circulating in your body. Just place your hands on the opposite shoulder and squeeze!

Move your hands down your arms and squeeze some more. You are worth holding onto! You are a gift! You are huggable and lovable! Additionally, sharing a hug and such a sentiment with someone else would be therapeutic for both of you I am sure.

The Power's in the Legs

"She's got legs—she knows how to use 'em!" The famous ZZ Top line rings true! We women love to flaunt our slim, trim legs. There is no song out there about our shapely arms. Let's face it, we women will rarely be able to outdo our male counterparts in upper body strength, but we certainly can look a lot better than them in a miniskirt. Recall the flopped attempt by the fashion industry in the nineties to stylize men's skirts. Not so pretty.

When it comes to outdoing a man in strength, there is the occasional exception such as the teenage female gymnast or softball pitcher, facing off against the cocky prepubescent male jock. Often this boy has a postpubescent ex-jock father who has unwittingly ingrained in his son's impressionable brain that males are the superior gender based on their upper body strength and lower body unique appendage. Just to give our boys the benefit of the doubt, however, an arm wrestling competition may be the only way they can figure out how to get physical contact with a girl. Or they may just be plain ignorant to the whole girl power idea and not even realize that it takes quite a few years until their testosterone will outdo the estrogen. But we all know where this is going. The girl humiliates him in a one-on-one arm wrestling competition and puts him in his place for a day or two.

Back to the point: Our power is in our lower extremities. If a woman needs to defend herself against a male of the aforementioned personage, she better use her legs. Her brains of course will also come in handy, which in my opinion the majority of the time females outdo their male counterparts in as well. The right brain typically tends to be a bit more dominant in the majority of females. This side of the brain is responsible for creativity and can help in thinking quickly in a tough situation, as long as their emotional brain doesn't paralyze them. Additionally I have observed an even more valuable tendency for women to be able to naturally develop both their right and left brains to look at situations holistically. Any of you typically left-brain dominant males out there who happen to be reading this—please do not misunderstand. I think there are many of you who incorporate your right brain quite well, but you have had to fight societal views and primitive ecology to do so. Kudos to you. And ladies, I sincerely hope you are appropriately grateful if you are married or attached to such a man or at least one with the humility to know his limitations.

Strong will and strong legs can thwart unwanted advances, especially one whose perpetrator is a drunk college boy who may, in his right mind, know that the female he is pursuing may be more impressed if he were in a sober state, or at least have a little more self-control and know what the two-letter word "No!" means. Even a potential rape can be interrupted by a woman with strong lower extremities. There is the classic knee to the groin, followed by a stomp on his foot, followed by running as fast as you can. Incidentally, the stomp on the instep can be even more effective if stilettos are the footwear of choice for that evening. High heels may make the sprinting part of the scenario a little more challenging however, but kicking them off before starting the sprint is always an option. Very strong adductors (these are the muscles, which squeeze ones thigh's together) can also come in handy as one reaches for a weapon of some sort to strike the perpetrator in the face with if advances progress to a point of danger. I in no way am meaning to make light of such a situation. Actually, I am attempting to do just the opposite.

Unfortunately, these methods are not always successful in thwarting a potential rape, and if anyone who is reading this has been in such a precarious situation, I want to say that whatever the outcome, it was not your fault. Some of the most mentally, emotionally and physically strong females have fallen prey to such horrendous attacks on our bodies and souls. Know you are not alone. Know it's okay to cry even if it happened thirty years ago.

There are many of us who have struggled for years and never told a soul about what happened because we blame ourselves or because we're embarrassed or because we just want to put it out of our minds. But the truth is, it is still there. It is a wounded part of you that maybe needs a little time and attention to fully heal. This part of your past may be negatively impacting current relationships and self-esteem. Your ability to be free of anxiety and to feel and express joy may be suffering. You may be struggling with parenting your teenage daughter or son effectively. The list really is endless. If through self introspection, you determine there is a part of your past that has left a festering wound in your soul, please don't ignore this history any longer.

Everyone will have a different way to work through the trauma. The great majority need a counselor to talk through things with: maybe a friend, maybe a family member, maybe a pastor, but most likely a professional counselor. My biggest advice though is to be gentle with yourself. That's really what this book is about—taking the time to do something for you—something that will help both your body and your soul.

Mentioning this very real and sad societal issue in this book, amidst its jocular and uplifting nature, is not done without much contemplation. I wish I could say that having strong legs could decrease your odds of having such a traumatic event in your life.

I wish I could say that having higher self-esteem, which often comes with exercising and taking better care of oneself, will help you avoid such awful situations. Unfortunately, life is full of suffering and there are no guarantees that anyone will be spared. But I do know this; recovering from the bruises and breaks of life is possible, and one likely will heal quicker if one practices self-care, both physically and emotionally.

Unfortunately, I speak from personal experience on such matters. The latest statistic, I have heard, is that one in every four women will experience abuse at some point in her life. It is not uncommon and tragically sad that women who are abused at a young age often experience similar or other forms of abuse in their later years. Why this is, I do not understand fully, I just know it to be true in my case and in many others. Fortunately, I have repressed many of the morbid details of my brief-yet-profoundly-painful encounter with a family friend of my youth. I still think about his children and can only pray that they broke the cycle of what was likely a very disturbed family line.

With a significant amount of counseling under my belt and ongoing hard work, I continue to grow into a strong, confident woman. I will always have scars from my past, but most of the pain is gone now. Occasionally I have a memory or an experience that flares up the old scar tissue and makes healing of new, seemingly insignificant wounds more difficult for me than another person without such a history may experience. We all heal at different rates. One of the worst things a person can say to someone, is "Why don't you just move on? Toughen up? Get over it?" etc. Often people that have suffered some affront in their past, don't even realize the impact it has on their healing potential for later psychological or physical traumas.

With the knowledge that even the most devastating trauma, be it to one person, or a whole community, be it physical or emotional, through nurturing, compassion, and patience, there can come healing and wholeness. Whatever a woman's past may be, there is nothing insignificant in life. All our experiences hold meaning and should not be minimized nor exaggerated. A small wound that is ignored can become a festering wound that leads to sepsis, potentially killing your body or soul without the proper care and attention. A seemingly insignificant wound that sets someone into a state of panic can result in devastating problems despite the proper medical attention. To a certain extent, it is up to the individual to determine how they will react to a trauma. What makes a person is not what happens in their life, but in essence how they respond to what happens in their life.

So let us embrace a positive response. Exercise is a way to release your body's natural painkillers known as endorphins. With the advent of amazing technology, power wheelchairs run by a puff of breath and computers controlled by eye gaze enable even a physically paralyzed person to no longer be trapped in a world of immobility and helplessness. Don't trap yourself in a world of emotional paralysis, immobility, and weakness simply by failing to adequately use the functioning neuromuscular system you possess. Weakness and immobility rarely happens overnight, just as a person's heart rarely is totally healthy one day and the next day no longer functioning. It is a slow gradual process toward dysfunction. Reversing that process only requires action. Initiation frequently precedes motivation. The motivation often will come after, not before you get moving!

We will be covering strengthening exercises for the gluts (more specifically the gluteus maximus, the gluteus medius, and the gluteus minimus if you like big words to throw around). We also will be addressing the quads and the hamstrings. For those of you aspiring physical therapists, I am now going to proudly give you the name of the quads with a little story along with.

Although I have worked in the medical field for over twenty years now, until recently, I often would feel intimidated by physicians, especially those of the male persuasion. I was quite empowered recently when I walked into the nursing station and one of our hospitalists (these are MDs who specialize in hospital care—a relatively new specialty) told another doctor on duty that day, "Ask her—she'll know." They could only remember one of the four quads. Now these are two of the smartest men I know—one a bit smarter than the other—the one who said to ask me. He's the medical director of the hospital for a reason—because he knows that his staff all have unique and helpful knowledge whether they are an MD with years of schooling or a housekeeper who knows where to find a certain supply.

So besides the rectus femoris which they remembered, I spouted off in two seconds flat, the vastus lateralis, the vastus medialis and the vastus intermedius. So the moral of this story ladies—be proud of your knowledge! Whether it's the names of muscles that nobody but us nerdy medical professionals are interested in, or it's the secret recipe for the scrumptious mint chocolate upside down cake for the annual New Year's Eve party!

Following is the biggest group of exercises I will review in any one chapter of this book. It is not necessary to do every exercise listed to address all the major muscle groups responsible for toning your buttocks and thighs. If you do one exercise from each of the six groups you will have a well balanced lower extremity workout. I also point out a couple different ways to combine exercises.

A good rule of thumb is ten to thirty repetitions of each exercise done slowly, counting from two to three for each movement. Personally, I'm not the type to count exercises and prefer to go until I begin to feel fatigued. If you are the type of person who likes to count or is very goal oriented and likes to note progress, I would recommend starting with ten or fifteen reps and upping the count five per exercise session. Once you feel little fatigue after thirty repetitions, then likely you need to proceed to a more challenging exercise. Also, I will offer modifications to make some exercises more or less challenging.

Hip Extensors–First Muscle Group

Many times I have heard woman complain about their flat bums. I really have to use all my restraint to not give them a lecture on exercise. So here is my chance! If you are tired of baggy pants, the first two muscle groups of these lower extremity exercises should not be skipped. What gives your rear its curves certainly has something to do with where one stores fat, but moreso, it has to do with how toned the muscles are below the fat.

Isometric Gluts or Glut Sets

There's really no picture necessary for this one as it is extremely basic. Isometric gluteal muscles sets is the technical name for butt squeezes, toosh tighteners, or get a beauty booty clenches. Basically squeeze your buttocks together, hold for a count of five, rest, repeat—as many times as you can until you feel the burn, get distracted, or die of boredom and need to move on. The nice thing about glut sets are they can be done in whatever position you happen to be in when you think of this exercise—not necessarily in the bathtub even—while your clothes shopping may be a particularly motivating opportunity or while you're watching "So You Think You Can Dance", "Survivor" or a myriad of other shows that make you just slightly jealous of the beautiful bodies you're being entertained by. Additionally this is a very inconspicuous exercise. It can be done sitting on the bus or waiting in line without anyone noticing, unless someone happens to be staring at your booty, and in that case, chances are you're making nice progress in your exercise routine—*Bravo* and *bum's the word!*

Bathtub Bridges:

This exercise also exercises the gluteals, but is a little more challenging than the above isometric exercise. There are two different variations to this exercise depending on your more comfortable starting position. Shorter individuals may prefer keeping feet on the base of the tub and taller people may choose keeping feet on the front ledge of the tub. If either method is comfortable, keep in mind the feet on the ledge offers a bit more of a challenge. If you have cervical issues a rolled up towel in the curve of your neck would be a good addition to this exercise. Take care not to put pressure against the back wall of the tub with your head, especially if your neck is bent.

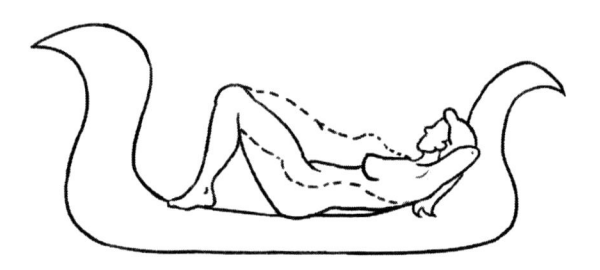

- Begin with your upper body floating or gently resting against the back of the tub and put your hand(s) behind your neck for support.
- Plant your feet firmly on the base of tub or ledge at the front of the tub with your knees bent.
- While pushing down with feet, lift your hips off base of tub and up toward water line. The goal is to eventually be able to lift your hips high enough so that your body is in a straight line from your knee caps to your upper trunk.
- Lower hips slowly and repeat.
- To make this exercise more challenging you may place your feet on the front ledge of the tub.
- If you still want more of a challenge lift one leg so the foot is suspended in the water or airborne and do a one legged bridge.

Hip Abductors–Second Muscle Group

Abductors is the technical word for muscles that spread the legs apart. The gluts are also responsible for this action. Most people have heard the bum muscles referred to as the gluts. What many don't know is there are three sets of gluts- the gluteus maximus, the gluteus medius and the gluteus minimus. The gluteus medius and minimus are the primary abductors while the gluteus maximus is the primary extensor which we exercised in the set before. All three muscles work together, but different ones take the lead or do the majority of the work depending on the action. I believe the abductors are one of the most important although neglected muscle groups in our lower extremities. Weak abductors are often the culprit in not only hip problems, but recent research is showing us that knee problems are often related to weak abductors as well.

Abductor Sets

This exercise is another example of an isometric muscle contraction in which we will use the walls of the bathtub for resistance. Sitting in an upright posture with straight legs, push both legs against the side walls of the bathtub. You can do this movement with your knees pointing straight up or turned outward slightly. If you tend to walk with your toes pointing inward I recommend trying to have your knees rotate out slightly with this exercise. If, on the other hand, you walk more like a duck, with your toes pointing out, try to keep your knee caps pointing toward the ceiling while you push against the walls of the tub. Hold the push for a count of five. Relax and repeat until you "feel the burn".

Incidentally, that burning sensation you feel is the buildup of lactic acid in your muscles and is a sign that you are pushing them sufficiently enough to create a chemical change in your muscles which will lead to new muscle growth as long as you don't push it too hard. Believe it or not, people (men in particular) have been known to land themselves in the hospital with a very serious medical condition called rhabdomyolysis (scary sounding word and yes it is) from overdoing it in a max lift muscle contraction. It is virtually impossible however to harm yourself significantly doing isometric muscle contractions.

Snow Angels

Wider tubs and jacuzzis are more effective to get the full benefit of this exercise. Nevertheless, this is an exercise that you can do mostly isometrically as outlined above and just add whatever movement your bathtub allows. In a semi- reclined position, spread your legs apart and then draw them together as if making angels in the snow like when you were a kid.

- Keep your toe pointing toward the ceiling to avoid muscle substitution and isolate the abductors more effectively.
- If you are in an extra large body of water you can simultaneously exercise your arms to make the angel wings while floating on your back.
- Repeat 10-30x.

This is a nice time to take a few deep breaths and connect with your guardian angel. If you have children you can also say protection prayers to your kids' guardian angels. Even though you may not see them, or hear them, sit quietly and have faith they are nearby, amongst the clatter and the noise, amongst the irritations and discouragements. Angels share their peaceful nature, lift you up with joyful presence, and cover you with their nurturing wings to keep you safe from the storms and foibles of daily life.

Adductors – Third Muscle Group

Opposite of abductors above, adductors squeeze the legs together.

Adductor sets

These are very similar to glut sets. Instead of tightening your buttocks, you tighten your inner thigh muscles, by pressing your thighs together. Hold 3-5 seconds. Relax. Repeat. You know the drill. You can do these simultaneously with the glut sets in any comfortable position, especially if you're short on time, but it is also good to learn how to isolate muscle groups.

Clam Shells

Clam shells actually strengthen a few muscle groups- adductors, abductors, internal and external rotators. Clam shells can be done lying on your back as well, but in the bath tub they are more effective for both range of motion and strengthening if done in sidelying.

- Turn onto your side and support your head with your forearm or hand depending on the water depth.

- Keeping your feet together, open and close your thighs, squeezing your knees together and then spreading them apart.
- Repeat 10-30x.
- Roll over and repeat 10-20x on the other side.

Hip Flexors–Fourth Muscle Group

Some of the muscles that cross the hip joint also cross the knee joint, so typically you will be exercising more than just one muscle group when doing the following exercises. When short on time you can skip the quadriceps exercises in muscle group five and just do the straight leg raise in this muscle grouping or skip the hamstring exercises in muscle group six and just do the heel slides below. Or you could do the straight leg raise and one hamstring exercise and cover three muscle groups. Get the idea? The more you get to know your body, the more you will be able to customize an exercise program that works for you.

Heel Slides

This very basic exercise is a nice warm up for stiff sore muscles and especially good if you have any limitations in the bending of your hip or knee. A person with good knee range of motion and body composition should be able to pull their heel to their bum and their knee to their chest. If you are a long ways off from that or have pain doing so, this exercise should always be included in your repertoire.

- Begin in a reclined position.
- Keep one leg straight.
- Keep the other leg's foot on the floor of the tub, and slide the foot along the base of the tub, toward the buttocks.
- Then straighten the leg and repeat 10-30x.
- Repeat with the opposite leg.
- Another option that incorporates a bit more abdominal activation and bilateral integration is to alternate your right and left leg so that while bending one leg you simultaneously straighten the other and repeat rhythmically as if pedaling a bike in the bathtub.

Straight leg raise

This exercise strengthens muscles from both the fourth muscle group and the fifth muscle group so if you are running short on time this is a good choice. It is also a pretty basic exercise, but a bit more difficult than the heel slide, especially if you have significant hip or knee weakness. If the straight leg raise is painful, which is a possibility in people with early hip arthritis, begin by getting stronger by doing extra repetitions of heel slides and hip abductor exercises outlined above. When you are ready for straight leg raises, modify the height of the leg lift so that it is pain free. If you have a deep bathtub, keeping the leg fully in the water may help as well.

- Start in a reclined position
- Keep one leg straight and the opposite leg bent with the sole of your foot on the base of your tub.
- Lift the straight leg up so that the foot comes out of the water.
- Hold for a count of 3-5 and lower slowly.
- Repeat 10-30x
- Repeat with opposite leg.

Quadriceps–Fifth Muscle Group

Quad Sets

Although the below picture shows the heels resting on the front ledge of the tub, this exercise can be done with your legs flat on the base of the tub as well. The advantage to doing the exercise with your knee joint airborne is that gravity can assist you in gaining terminal knee extension. This is the last five to ten degrees of knee extension, often referred to as hyperextension. This movement is often the first range we loose in an arthritic or traumatically damaged knee. Regaining this range can mean the difference between suboptimal and fully functioning knee joints.

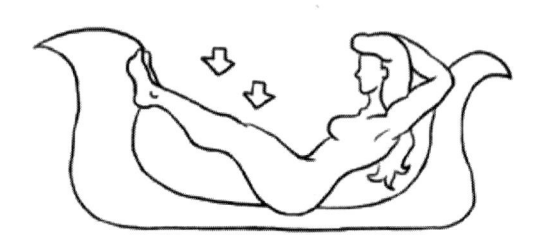

- Begin in a reclined position.
- Place hand(s) behind head or neck for optimal neck support.
- Rest your ankles on the front ledge of the tub or flat on the base of the tub.
- Tighten the muscles on the front of your thighs as if you are trying to push your knee cap down into the water.
- Hold for a count of 3-5 seconds.
- Repeat 10-30 times.

If you exercise both the knees simultaneously, you may notice some slight asymmetry in your ability to get that full amount of extension. This is really nothing to be alarmed about especially if there is no pain involved. We are all a bit asymmetrical. But this does sometimes indicate early arthritic changes. Continuing with a good exercise program for your knees will be important for your ongoing health and comfort.

Long Arc Quads

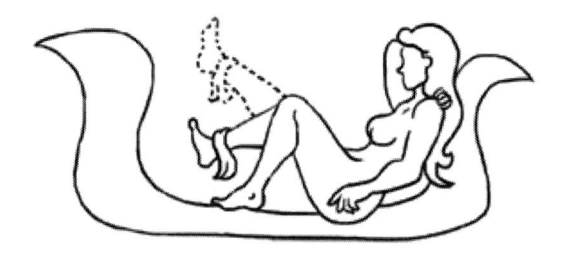

- Begin in a supported reclined position.
- Cross the right leg over the left leg for additional support, or stabilize the right leg by pressing your right thigh against the left thigh.
- Fully straighten and bend the right knee.
- Repeat until fatigued
- Repeat with the left leg.
- Add a wet towel draped over your ankle for extra weight as needed.

Hamstrings- Sixth Muscle Group

I have found the hamstrings to be the most challenging muscle group to exercise effectively in the bathtub. Likely this is due to the fact that these four different muscles like their counterbalancers, the quads, are an extremely strong group of muscles.

There is another more effective option in the shower sequel chapter and the hamstrings are also exercised in coordination with other muscles during some of our core activities in the next chapter.

Hamstring Curls

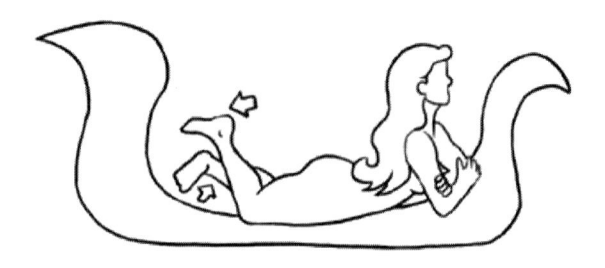

- Roll onto your stomach and prop on elbows. Cross your arms in front if needed to allow for sufficient room in the tub.
- Cross your legs at your ankles.
- Bend your knees fully and straighten.
- After a few repetitions, apply slight downward pressure from the leg resting on top onto the lower leg while lifting the lower leg upward.
- Repeat 10–30x.
- Cross your legs in the opposite direction and apply pressure downward while lifting upward on the opposite leg.
- Repeat 10–30x.

- If this is slightly awkward, you may try using a wet towel for resistance. However this can be awkward as well as the towel tends to slip.

Whew—lots of exercises there! Good Job! Sorry if I got a bit carried away, but PTs love legs. What I have seen in my twenty-some-year career is that people that keep moving, keep grooving. The single most important factor I have seen that is attached to quality of life as people age is their ability to keep physically fit. Most people just take for granted what a blessing it is to be able to walk. I have known many people, by no fault of their own, who either never had or lost the ability to walk. However, I have also known some who lose the ability to walk due to their own self neglect or self abuse over the years. So count your blessings now and do what it takes to keep yourself healthy and strong and walking on a regular basis as long as you possibly can.

If you lead a sedentary lifestyle, it can be an almost imperceptibly slow decline to becoming deconditioned if you do not begin to push yourself . However, it is not difficult to gradually engage in more rigorous activity. You have already begun a new habit with you tub exercises. The next step may be a morning or lunchtime walk, a weekend hike, or an evening of mall walking- whichever steps seem more in sync with your rhythm of life.

Tummy Time

At the Center of it all is your abdominal muscles, lovingly referred to as the *abs* or the *pooch*. The decision is yours. You can have a pooch and just lumber along, not necessarily having a weak body, but certainly not having the body you need to reach your utmost potential. Or you can have abs of steel and meet challenges with strength and fortitude. Getting to the core of the issue is imperative when dealing with any problem in life or with your body. Often a musculoskeletal issue can be traced back to core muscle weakness.

Mental health issues tend to be the same way. If you don't get to the core of why you behave in self-destructive ways and do the hard work it takes to change behaviors, get stronger, and experience healing, chances are you're going to struggle much more in solving your issues and growing into the person God designed you to be. Getting to the core of problems can be painful, but it is usually necessary to find a solution. Exercising the core muscles is the most challenging of workouts, but also brings about the most benefit.

If I was asked to label an area of the body that, as a PT, I am passionate about, it would be the tummy. And with pediatrics being one of my favorite populations to work with, that is the terminology I would use. Around the turn of the century when the "Back to Sleep" movement arose, we noticed an interesting trend in pediatrics. In the early 1990s, parents were told to place their newborns on their stomachs to sleep most safely. By the mid-nineties, we were told side-lying was the safest position and there was a massive amount of commercialized infant side-lying positioners sold that rarely held a wiggling ball of energy in that position longer than a couple hours at best. By the year 2000, when my last child was born, there was some anecdotal evidence that the highest rate of occurrence of SIDS deaths was found when infants were sleeping on their stomachs and the "Back to Sleep" movement was started by the medical community. Unfortunately, this created an unduly large amount of anxiety in new parents about placing children on their tummies at all, even when awake.

The pediatric therapy community noticed delays in otherwise healthy babies in their gross motor skills, due at least in part to infants and babies not given adequate time to explore their environment on their bellies so they didn't learn to roll or crawl at a standard rate. Additionally, there was an increase in cranial abnormalities, with babies developing abnormally flat skulls from always having pressure on the backs of their heads. This had to do with not only sleeping on their backs, but the vast amount of time spent in car seats, swings, vibrating/bouncy chairs, etc. which all positioned babies on their backs. So the medical community had to follow up the "Back to Sleep" movement with the "Tummy Time" movement.

Although tummy time was developed for little ones, I am also a proponent for tummy time for us aging bodies. This can help to keep your spine in good alignment, improve shoulder range of motion and strength and helps to take pressure off of bulging disks. Tummy time is also incorporated into my bathtub exercises. You simply roll onto your stomach and prop on your elbows. This may be an awkward position for you initially. In that case, you may need to spend a couple weeks just lying on your stomach on your bed or the floor. Then focus on the prone (stomach) on elbows position before advancing to prone push-ups.

Likely, the majority of you have experienced back pain at some point in your life. If you haven't yet, chances are you will. The reason for this epidemic is multifactorial in my opinion. One of the contributing factors is the all-or-none mentality of many in our society. More and more people are leading a sedentary lifestyle as technology has come to dominate our world. With that sedentary lifestyle comes less and less natural opportunities to strengthen and stretch the spinal complex. Then people go to do something fun like hit the slopes on the weekend, play a round of golf, decide they're going to get in shape and start with a ninety-minute Zumba class, or simply bend over to pick up a box and there goes the back. Gaining and maintaining spinal flexibility and core strength are imperative to decreasing your odds that you will injure your back. If you are physically and mentally healthy, and experience a back issue anyway, the greater the odds will be that you can rehab quickly and your back pain will not become a chronic problem or one that limits your function.

The spine is made up of twenty-four stacking vertebrae and twenty-four disks. Each vertebra has essentially eight different joints. There are literally hundreds of muscles, tendons, ligaments, and nerves that are susceptible to wear and tear and injury in your spine. So do the math. There are a multiplicity of potential problems. However, there are also a multiplicity of amazing things that can be done with a body due to the flexibility of the spine. I have witnessed this in awe as I have watched my youngest flip and twirl her way around the gymnastic apparatus, my middle dive to stop a soccer ball coming at him sixty miles per hour, or my eldest take a shot on goal with the power of a 5'11" male, rather than a 5'2" teenage girl. The abilities, determination, and beauty of the human body constantly amaze me, especially as I am watching one of my children.

Unfortunately though, as we age, the effects of gravity and years of either neglect or wear and tear can take their toll. We either wear out or rust out. In my opinion wearing out is the better of these two options but the third option of having a balanced body is the ideal. Besides kyphosis (the forward curvature or hunching over we often see as we age), which we combat with tummy time, there are some other not-so-pleasant possibilities to potentially experience in the aging process. Those of you who have gone through a pregnancy are likely familiar with Kegel exercises. Neglect of this exercise during and after this period of life can lead to some embarrassing incidents, or shall we say accidents, especially when jumping or sneezing is involved.

For those of you who are a bit perplexed right now, basically Kegels are a contraction of your pelvic floor muscles. It involves actively contracting the muscles surrounding your urethral and vaginal outlet (fondly referred to by many a potty training parent as the pee-pee hole). Of course the anatomy is obviously different in little boys and little girls, but we have the same three muscles that contract or relax, typically without too much active thought to control the flow or urine.

There are numerous other muscles of the pelvic floor anatomy, which most physical therapists don't even know or care to know the names of. So we will not get any more detailed in the explanation. However, I must say this is one of the easiest muscles to exercise, because no matter where you are or what you are doing, if you are fully clothed, and honestly, even if you're not, someone would have to be very up close and personal to know you are contracting these muscles.

Kegels

- Relax in any position in the tub.
- Squeeze your pelvic floor muscles as if you're trying to not pee in your pool.
- Hold for a count of 3-5.
- Fully relax and repeat.

A close relative to the Kegel exercise is the pelvic tilt. This is the most important exercise in this chapter. If you can learn how to perform a good pelvic tilt this will put you miles ahead in your journey toward gaining a strong core. The lower abdominals are the most difficult to strengthen and at the same time the most important to safeguard against low back injury.

Pelvic Tilt

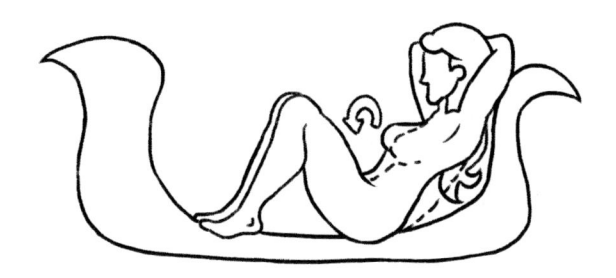

- Lie in a reclined position or flat on the base of your tub with knees bent.
- Rock your pelvis forward as if there is a string pulling your belly button upward toward your nose. If you are doing this correctly you should feel your low back begin to flatten.
- Hold your back flat against the base of the tub for 3-5 seconds then relax.
- Repeat 10-30x until you feel the burn in the muscles in the area under your navel.

Some of the exercises following will refer to the pelvic tilt as a component. So it is important to solidify this exercise. Although to some this may seem very simple, others may find it very challenging. I will never forget when a classmate jumped up on the lecture demo table one of the last days of PT school and proudly demonstrated his beautiful pelvic tilt. It was hilarious. But it honestly took him nearly two years to perfect this exercise because he was so bound down and unable to move his pelvis efficiently at the beginning of grad school. Now that you have learned the pelvic tilt we can move onto the standard abdominal exercises.

For those of you familiar with the classic sit-up, I must tell you that the majority of people do it incorrectly if the desire is to strengthen the core. The pairing up of partners at the instruction of physical education teachers is a valid technique for providing motivation to a buddy. However, by having the ankles held down, typically hip flexors are utilized more than the abdominals.

There are four sets of abdominal muscles. The classic sit-up focuses on one of the four: the much sought-after *six-pack* or rectus abdominis. Actually, in the most lean and toned elite athletes, you can often see an eight-pack. The *rectus*, however, as appealing as it may be, is not the most important abdominal muscle for core strength, as it serves primarily one purpose, trunk flexion.

There are many other core muscles that can be unintentionally neglected by those who choose to do only the classic sit-up, which I will cover, albeit a bit modified as tummy tucks.

If doing all of the core exercises listed below during your first few sessions feels overwhelming, that's okay. One should to not take on too much too soon. Just vary which ones you do so that you do not neglect a certain muscle group. Or just do a few repetitions of all of them and work on slowly increasing the number of reps. Remember there's more to core than tummy tucks!

Crunches/ Tummy Tucks

- Begin lying on your back, with upper trunk buoyant and knees bent.
- Perform a pelvic tilt.
- Supporting your neck with your hands, raise your chest up out of the water line so that

your hips and knees are bent to about a 45 degree angle.
- Lower. Rest and Repeat

So with crunches we exercise about twenty five percent of our abdominals. Now it's time to address the other seventy five percent. While the rectus performs trunk flexion or bending, the other three abdominal muscles are primarily responsible for trunk rotation, compression, and elongation. The internal and external obliques, and the transverse abdominis are the technical names. A good personal trainer, physical therapist, physical education teacher, athletic trainer or coach should never neglect "the obliques" which these three muscles are often grouped together as. They certainly will not be neglected here.

Tucks With a Twist

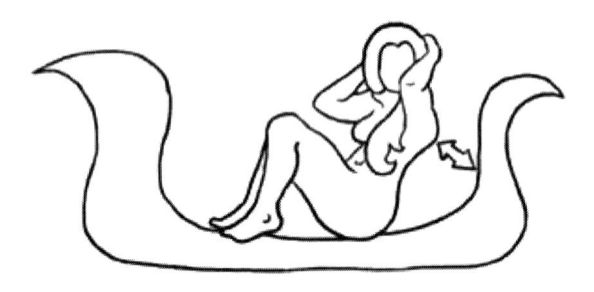

- Begin lying on your back, with upper trunk reclined or buoyant and knees bent.
- Perform a pelvic tilt.

- Supporting your neck with your hands, raise yourself up, directing your right elbow toward your left knee.
- If you desire a little more movement in your hips and/or trunk, place your left ankle on your right knee then bring your right elbow to your left knee.
- Lower, rest and repeat.

Before changing positions you can try "the slides". They use the principle of the smooth frictionless bathtub so it may not work as well for you if you have texture on the base of your tub. Do these exercises very slowly or you may have a mini flood to mop up. Additionally, by going slowly you will get the most benefit from these exercises which work a variety of muscles in conjunction. They probably are the most difficult of this chapter.

Push Pull Slide

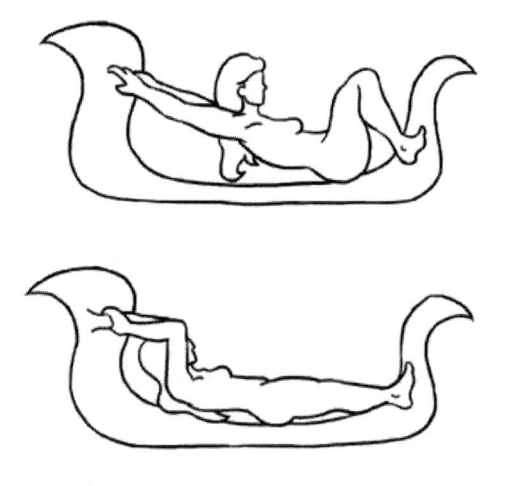

- Position yourself in the center of the tub and recline with your head near the front rather than the back of the tub.
- Grab the Spigot over your head and pull yourself toward the spigot careful not to bump your head, straightening your legs while bending your arms.
- Perform a pelvic tilt to activate your core.
- Continue to hold onto the spigot.
- Then straighten your arms while simultaneously bending your legs, sliding your body toward the back wall of the tub.
- Repeat the above sequence 10-30x.

With this exercise you can focus more on pulling with your upper body or pushing with your lower body to slide, whichever feels more natural or needs more work. Additionally, to work the obliques a bit more in the slide exercises, let your legs drop slightly to one side or the other when the knees are bent. Also, especially if you have a wider tub, you can slide your body in diagonals rather than straight planes.

Sit Up Slide

This is a bit more abdominal work than its predecessor "The Slide." To give your core a better workout do the below sequence very slowly and in between movements take your feet off the ledge of the tub and hold for a count of three to five.

The Dizzy Woman's Bathtub Guide

- Lay in the tub with your head relaxing in the water.
- Your legs should be straight and resting on the front ledge of the bathtub or the wall above the bathtub.
- Bend your shoulders and elbows.
- Place your wrists next to your ears and your palms on the back wall of the bathtub.
- Push off with your hands so that as you straighten your elbows your body slides toward the front ot the tub and your legs bend.
- Once your arms are straight, lift them straight toward the ceiling.

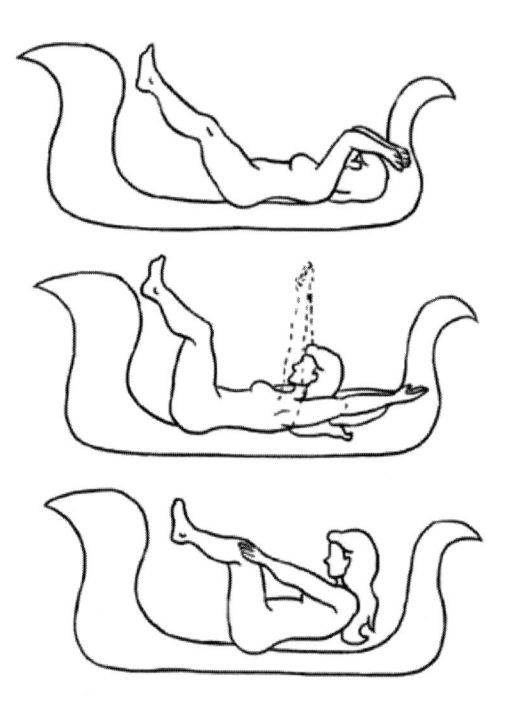

- Then lift your torso, keeping your arms nearly in the same position until your hands touch your knees.
- Lower your torso slowly.
- Place your feet on the front wall of the tub and push back slowly by straightening your legs until your head reaches the back wall of the tub reaching back with your arms to avoid bumping your head.
- You should now be back near the starting position.
- Repeat the sequence 10-30x.

This exercise may seem a bit complicated, but try not to overthink it. Basically, rather than pulling with your arms like in the "Push Pull Slide", you are pushing and adding a sit up between pushing with your arms and pushing with your legs. Now, before rolling into prone, there are a couple exercises to be done in sidelying.

Quad Stretch

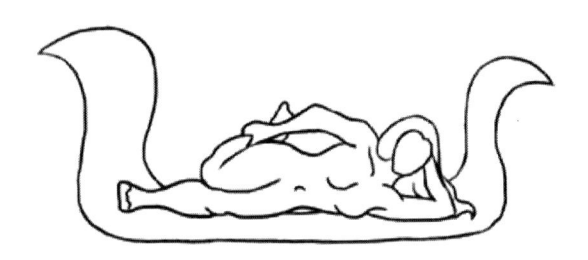

- Lie on your right side with both legs slightly bent and the lower arm supporting your head/neck.
- Bend your left leg a little more and grab your ankle with your left hand, palm on the bony prominence on the outside of your left ankle.
- Then gently pull your left foot towards your buttocks.
- Hold for a count of 30-60 seconds.
- Relax.
- Roll onto your left side and repeat the stretch with your right leg.

Sidelying situps

This exercise focuses on your quadratus lumborum. I've always loved that name for some reason, so I'm sharing it with you anatomical terminology fans. It is a large muscle that basically attaches your pelvis to your low back.

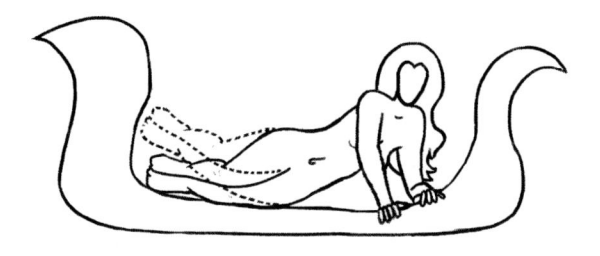

- Lie on your left side with both legs slightly bent and the left arm supporting your head/neck or propping on the base of the tub.
- Your right arm should be placed on the tub in front of your belly to provide a bit of leverage.
- Raise both legs up simultaneously just out of the water.
- Lower and repeat 10-30x as able.
- Roll to the opposite side and repeat.
- After you can perform 30 reps relatively easily, you may try raising your torso simultaneously with raising legs for an extra challenge.

Now it's tummy time! Lying on your stomach in the bathtub may seem a strange thing to do, but it is actually very relaxing as well as good for your spine. If all you do is rest on your elbows for a few minutes on the first attempt, that is a fine start. Just work on your deep breathing exercises in this position until you feel more comfortable.

Prone Pushups

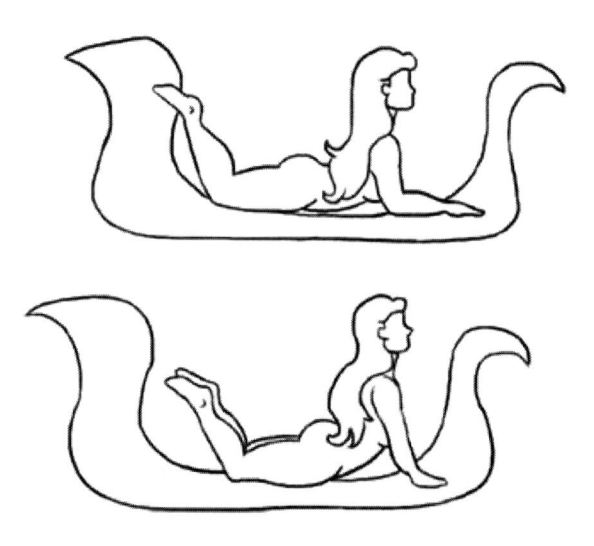

- Lie on your stomach with your forearms on the base of the tub and your knees slightly bent so shins/ankles rest on back ledge of tub or remain relaxed in an air born position.
- While keeping your pelvis firmly on the base of the base of the tub, straighten your elbows as far as comfortably possible while arching your back.
- Hold for a count of 5-10 seconds.
- Repeat 5-15x.

The Bathtub Plank

On land, a plank is typically done balancing on your forearms and your toes. However, unless you are below average height or your bathtub is above average length, it will likely be necessary to balance on your forearms and knees. If it is typically uncomfortable to be on your knees this may not be a problem with this exercise due to the pressure alleviation of the water. However, if it is, simply fold up your wet bath towel from previous exercises and lie it below your knees.

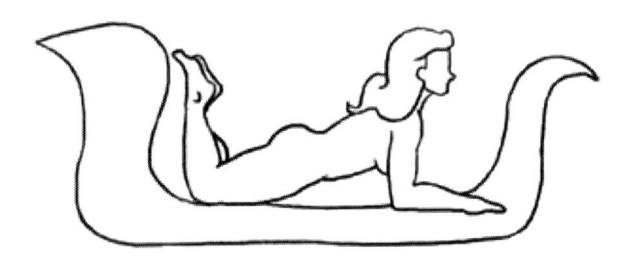

- Lie on your stomach with your forearms on the base of the tub and your knees slightly bent so shins/ankles rest on back ledge of tub or rest air born, crossing at the ankles for stability if needed.
- Stabilize your shoulder girdle and lift your pelvis off the base of the tub.
- Activate your abdominals by performing a pelvic tilt and flattening your back while you lift.

- Your goal is to have a straight diagonal line from the base of your neck to your knees.
- Attempt to hold this position as long as possible. A good indicator of being a physically fit individual is to be able to hold this plank for about 90 seconds.
- Repeat 3-10x.

Prone Hip extension

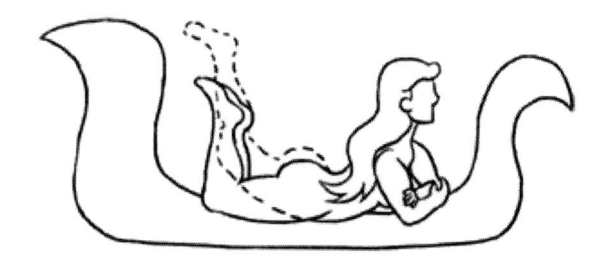

- Rest in the prone on elbows position, crossing your arms if needed to allow for more space.
- Bend your knees to an approximately 90 degree angle.
- Lift your entire leg up, maintaining the bent knee as if there is a string around your foot pulling it to the ceiling.
- Repeat 10-30x with the opposite leg.

If any of these prone exercises elicit back pain, maintain a pelvic tilt prior to performing the exercise and see if that helps.

I feel compelled to end this chapter discussing pain a bit more since many of these exercises are commonly prescribed for back pain. Back pain is one of the biggest reasons for absenteeism from work and frequently can lead to disability. It is therefore a significant issue in our society.

I believe there are many incidents of back pain for which the etiology or cause is not easily diagnosed or identified. In such cases treatment can be a challenge, and my issues certainly fell into that category. There are many related issues that often complicate back pain. Often our medical doctors, in their attempts to alleviate pain will prescribe medications. This is sometimes appropriate, but often risky in my opinion. Alleviating pain should certainly be a goal. But pain is a symptom, not a disease or condition. Determining the reason for the pain in my opinion is more important than masking discomfort if one's goal is to have lasting relief.

Getting to the core of the issue should always be the goal in trying to help someone who is struggling or suffering. That someone could be *yourself* either now or in the future. The pain experienced may be physically or emotionally based. Taking medications that mask physical symptoms can be problematic. Often dealing with some level of acute pain is part of the healing process in the case of musculoskeletal injury. People tend to be more careful in what they do and curtail their activities so they don't exacerbate the problem further if they are in a certain amount of pain.

Whether pain has a relatively benign orthopedic source or something more dangerous needs to be determined. So if you ever experience even relatively mild physical pain lasting more than a few days, be sure you are evaluated by a physician to rule out any serious causes. Be aware though, that often with back, neck, and extremity pain, the musculoskeletal system will be pegged as the culprit and often anxiety-driven muscle tension can be at the core of the problem. The more anxious one becomes about the pain or a crisis gong on in their life, the more muscle tension is created, and the pain then worsens, creating a vicious cycle. As difficult as it may seem, when you're hurting, it is important to stay as calm and relaxed as possible. If medication is needed to do this, then I would advise to cautiously take what is recommended. Just avoid becoming overly reliant on pharmaceuticals.

If someone takes strong pain medication, such as narcotics that only treat the symptoms and not the cause, the problem could get worse and often result in creating more issues. Narcotic drug addiction is an epidemic in this country. Whether medications are being prescribed by a physician or people are self-medicating with legal or illegal drugs, developing a drug addiction is a frightening risk often due to attempts to mask physical and/or emotional pain.

Whatever the issue, the cause should be treated, not just the symptom. Treating only the symptom can be like putting bandages over an infected wound. Just because you cannot see the problem, does not mean it's not there. As the bacteria multiply, the wound and the bandages you're covering them with just get bigger. Ironically, the bandage often will even make the environment more conducive to growing the bacteria. The infection won't go away until it is treated with antibiotics. Pain medication works much the same way. Sometimes the *wound* just gets bigger as you're attempting to cover it up with the *bandage* of pain meds. Obviously there are times when pain medication is imperative for healing, especially when the injury is severe and acute. Certain pain medicines can also quickly interrupt a pain/spasm/pain cycle or an inflammation process. Still however, if the core issue is more complicated, treatment with pain medication alone will usually not bring about healing.

There are also times during social/emotional crisis that covering up a problem while it just becomes more dangerous is not a wise strategy. Identifying the problem and facing it head on is usually necessary. Our neurological system may send us into a fight-or-flight mode in such cases. Fighting however is not always wise or productive, especially if you are a female, and physical threats are involved. We usually will lose.

So if you're in the middle of a war zone without any weapons for self-defense, and peace talks have failed, escaping the area may be the only way to protect yourself and those you love. Once in a safe place, healing can begin. Leaving a bad situation does not mean you are giving up, it can be just the opposite. It can mean you are saving yourself. One may choose to stay away permanently or temporarily. One may choose to return when the danger passes. In some cases, there may not be a home to return to, but as long as there has truly been a cease-fire and return is safe, homes and hearts can be rebuilt.

Shower Sequel

I realize that sometimes the practicality of the shower will win out over the bathtub. There are just some mornings that the only shot at getting sufficiently invigorated to move ahead with the day is to stumble into the shower and just stand there, allowing the life-giving force of the water to energize a halfway-sleeping body. Sometimes standing can even be too much!

I can remember during the depths of depression, waking up some mornings, utterly exhausted by a fitful, restless night that I would actually sit in the corner of my shower until I had the energy to stand. Sometimes, on a particularly bad day, that would be once the hot water heater was drained. Once the water got tepid, I knew I didn't have long before I would have to get moving or get really cold. Remember the Krebs cycle—movement creates energy, not the other way around.

Many of the exercises mentioned in this book, especially the upper body exercises, can easily be done in standing. The *shaving stretches* can also be easily done in standing. When shaving your legs, just focus on tightening up those quads and keeping your knee straight. Whether you are resting your heel on a shower seat or the edge of the tub or bending over at the hips, tightening the knee and bending at the hip rather than the spine will help to get an efficient hamstring stretch.

Postural correctness is just as important in standing as in sitting: Shoulders back, chin tucked, spine straight, abdominals activated, and knees straight, but not locked. Spend a bit of time as well focusing on your feet. Are your toes pointing straight ahead, not excessively in or out? Minimize toe curling, but attempt to have contact with all five toes. For that matter, attempt to assure you are bearing weight in a balanced manner throughout your foot. The weight on the heel and the ball of the foot should be relatively equal. The weight on the outside and inside of the foot should be equalized as well. Actually, concentrating on good posture for a few minutes and practicing deep diaphragmatic breathing (Refer to chapter two "Bathing for Beginners") can be a peaceful way to begin your day.

I could probably write a whole other book on an exercise routine to be done in the shower, but I will refrain for the time being and just give you a couple additional exercises that would help to complete your exercise program. The few exercises

I'm going to give you focus on muscles that are often difficult to stretch or strengthen sufficiently in the tub, especially as you get in better shape. However, I warn that if you are advanced in years or you have a history of balance issues, you should have a sturdy grab bar to support you for the exercises of this chapter. Even our younger counterparts who may be participating, be sure you start these exercises with a hand on the wall at least.

Heel Cord Stretch

This exercise will be important and should preceed *Toe Lifts*, especially if one finds that following exercise challenging.

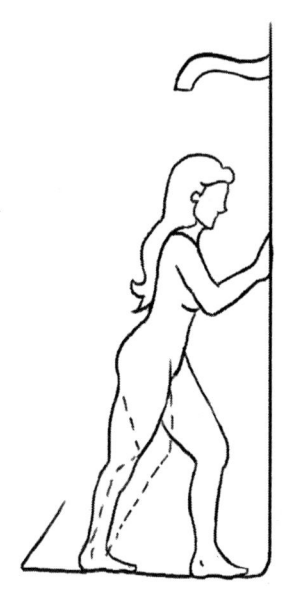

- Place your hands on the shower wall and both your feet about three feet away from the wall.
- Bring one foot forward.
- Keeping the forward knee slightly bent and the back leg straight, lunge forward pressing into the wall while keeping the heels flat and your back knee straight.
- You should feel the stretch in the calf belly of the straight leg in the back.
- After holding this position for thirty to sixty seconds, slightly bend the knee of the straight leg in back and hold again.
- You should now feel the stretch lower down in the calf, closer to the Achilles tendon. This muscle (the soleus—close cousin to the more universally known gastrocnemius or *gastrocs*) is often neglected when stretching out the calf muscle.
- Switch leg positions and repeat on opposite side.

Heel Lifts

- Hold onto the shower wall or a grab bar for support.
- Keep your knees and hips as straight as possible.

- Raise up onto tiptoes and then lower self slowly.
- Repeat 10-30x
- If this seems too simple and/or you want to further challenge your balance, attempt this exercise balancing on one foot while you raise up onto your tiptoe. Be sure you use hand support at least initially, no matter how in shape you think you are.

Toe Lifts

This tends to be a difficult task for some people. If you find yourself, sticking your bum out excessively while you attempt to do this exercise, chances are you have tight heel cords and/or weak shin muscles. If that's the case, preceeding this exercise with the Heel Cord Stretch explained above may help. This exercise should be more of a challenge if you focus on keeping your hips tucked in and your spine straight.

- Pull your toes up so your toes and the ball of your foot are off the shower floor surface and all your weight is on your heels.
- Hold for a count of three.
- Repeat 10–30x.

Squats

This is the classic weight bearing exercise to strengthen the Quadriceps. Of course in a weight bearing position there is more stress on the joints so those of you with arthritic knees need to be cautious to not squat too far initially– no buckling knees allowed! It is easier to make this exercise more challenging–just squat further down! Without hand support or lifting my heels up my knees can bend about forty-five degrees repetitively on a good day. When I am in an arthritic flare I may only squat about twenty degrees, at least for the first few repetitions, and either way there is a lot of snap crackle pop going on. Joint sounds are not necessarily a bad thing, but you should not push into pain during this exercise.

- Begin in good standing posture with feet aligned shoulder width apart, toes pointing straight ahead and weight distributed evenly throughout foot.
- Maintaining an upright trunk posture, slowly bend knees and hips.
- Strive to keep kneecaps pointing straight ahead while bending, not allowing knees to collapse inward or outward.
- Squat down as far as comfortable and slowly return to upright stance while maintaining your knee alignment.
- Repeat 10-30x.

Stork Stance:

Just balancing on one foot can also be a good exercise for both ankle strength and balance. Attempt to not let your arch collapse when you do this and keep your toes and knees pointing straight ahead. Many people collapse inward or outward at their knee or hip in one legged stance. So be sure you keep your knee aligned with the knee cap pointing straight ahead and do not allow your pelvis to drop down on the side of the airborn leg. Remember to use hand support for safety. Once you can do this activity with ease and feel well balanced for 20-30 seconds, you may then proceed to the next exercise. Otherwise save hamstring curls for once you have felt an improvement in your balance and pelvic strength.

Hamstring Curls

This is very similar to the exercise done in prone in "The Power's in the Legs" chapter except you should be able to work through your full range of motion against gravity. A towel ankle weight (the wetter the heavier) may still be needed if you find 20- 30 repetitions too easy.

- Begin in good standing posture, with one hand on the wall or a sturdy support handle.
- Lift one leg up.
- Keeping thigh in the vertical position, draw your foot up toward your buttocks.
- Squeeze for a count of 3-5, then slowly lower to the base of the shower.
- Assure you are fully balanced between and during repetitions and repeat 10-30x.
- Repeat with opposite leg.

The last exercise I will include can easily be done when rinsing your hair. Instead of just looking up with your neck to wet the crown of your head, extend your entire spine. Place your hands on both sides of your low back, right above your pelvis, then arch not only your neck, but your mid and low back as well. This will help to realign your vertebrae and discs that are typically over flexed throughout the day. Performing this maneuver a few times in a row frequently when getting out of the car or taking a standing break after sitting in front of a computer screen is a great idea as well. In theses cases you can just imagine the refreshing water as you take some deep breaths.

Water has the ability to either refresh or relax, cool or heat. A comfy water bed can lull you to sleep as if in the hull of a sailboat in a gentle harbor or a white water raft trip can give you the thrill of a lifetime. Water is as awe inspiring as gazing out along the ocean's horizon wondering at the mysteries within, and as pure as a drop of rain caught in the palm of a young child's hand.

Water nourishes a parched and thirsting body and soul. Water cleanses and heals, bringing us into new life. Grass stains or mud and blood from a skinned knee can be washed away by the water, just like the residue of our sins are washed away by the holy waters of Christ in baptism. Whether in a hot tub or a refreshing shower, immersing oneself in water at the day's beginning or end can help you to be reminded of the purity and holiness of water, and draw oneself to prayerful, peaceful time when we can simply listen and be still. Such time in this hectic world is so rare yet so needed to restore the mind, body and spirit.

Prayer can be a fountain of tranquility to those who seek it as such. Most of us make petitions sometimes without even realizing we are asking for God's help and intervention. Prayers of gratefulness and thanksgiving are sadly somewhat less common. But likely the most underutilized method of prayer and my personal savior is the contemplative form. In this we strive to listen to God, to hear his word and will spoken sweetly within our inner self and to feel the unspeakable peace that only union with our Lord and Savior can bring.

Finally the Feat

Although this chapter will be focusing on exercises for the feet, no, I have not misspelled the title. Because you are getting closer to the end of this book, and anyone who can listen to my incessant rambling on about the human body and soul while simultaneously participating in an exercise program while getting one's body squeaky clean and relaxed has accomplished a tremendous feat in my opinion. But what next? What is the next feat that is in store for you? I would like to suggest using your feet in other places rather than resting them up in a recliner chair or sitting them underneath a computer desk, or yes, even soaking them in a bathtub.

Remember it's all about balance—balancing activity and inactivity, balancing music to your ears and the sound of silence, balancing high expectations with tolerance and patience, balancing love of life and humility of spirit. If your life is out of balance in the area of aerobic activity, I would like to suggest that you hit the ground running with those beautiful feet of yours—or jogging, or walking, or sauntering—whichever fits your feet best. If you tend to be out of balance in the area of peacefulness, then taking up meditation, Tai Chi or Yoga would be highly recommended.

When you go to get that pedicure that you promised yourself you would do once you consistently did your exercise program a few times per week, I would recommend not driving around for ten minutes at the mall finding the closest parking space. Try instead parking in the first spot you see, no matter how far away and hoofing it. Research has shown that five to ten minutes of exercise interspersed randomly throughout the day makes a positive impact on cardiovascular health.

If you really want to shed pounds, better yet leave your car at home altogether and walk or bike to the nearest mall. Twenty minutes of aerobic exercise, at least four times weekly will make an impact and speed up that metabolism that slows to an alarming rate in sedentary individuals, woman over forty in particular. I have personally experienced this perimenopausal phenomenon and believe me the situation can quite quickly get out of hand if one fails to be proactive.

The following exercises are so simple that no pictures are required. However, although they are basic, sometimes it is the basics in life, the simplest things that we leave out, which can lead to our whole person being out of balance. Balance is unmistakably a complex concept which can be divided into three separate but equally important parts.

Great things come in threes! My kids of course are a given. But at a deeper level and one that applies to anyone, I believe that a truly whole person not only takes care of her body, but her mind and spirit as well. Body-Mind-Spirit: a beautiful threesome. In nature, we see the simple-yet-beautiful trillium flower. For those of you of Irish descent, there is of course the shamrock. Who doesn't love St. Patrick's Day? Green is a worldwide theme that we all need to pay more attention to. Many people don't understand the origins of this holiday, but Saint Patrick used the shamrock to explain the trinity to convert the Pagans of Ireland to Christianity. The Father, the Son, and the Holy Spirit—separate but the same, like the leaves of the shamrock. So simple yet so profound.

Back to the threefold nature of balance. Physiologically, your vision, inner ear, and proprioception are the three keys to balance. Proprioception fits into our sensory system under the sense of touch. We have these little *feeler cells* connected with our nerves and muscle cells that help to determine where your body is in space and make the proper adjustments to keep it upright. When you are standing, your feet are where the connection with the ground is happening and hence your ability to keep upright is largely reliant on your feet's ability to sense and make adjustments as needed. Strong, flexible feet are imperative to having good balance. There are also three types of balance reactions—ankle-foot reactions, knee-hip reactions, and protective stepping reactions.

There will be three (what a coincidence) foot exercises in this chapter. The muscles strengthened in the first two exercises are also the focus of a couple exercises mentioned in the "Shower Sequel" chapter. The exercises done standing in the shower will challenge your balance a bit more, but strengthening your foot and ankle muscles lying in the bathtub should also positively impact your balance, albeit indirectly.

- *First,* with your knees straight and legs resting on the base of the tub, simply bend your ankles so that your toes move toward your head. Pull them back as far as possible, keeping your knees straight, so you feel a gentle stretch in your calves. Hold for a count of three and repeat ten to thirty times.

- *Second,* also with your knees straight and legs resting on the base of the tub, point your feet as far as possible, tippy-toe style in honor of our inner ballerinas! This exercise can be done in the air or water to get the most range of motion possible or for more strengthening you can use the front wall of the tub for resistance by pushing your foot into the tub wall as if to point, but the wall of the tub will stop your movement. Either way, hold for a count of three and repeat ten to thirty times.

- *The third exercise* is a little twist on a classic physical therapy prescription for a recovering ankle sprain. The classic exercise (if you wish to do a monotonous activity) is to write the alphabet with your feet. By doing this, you are working all your foot muscles. We talked earlier in the book about trunk rotation being the key to strong abdominals. Well, foot rotation is the key to strong ankles and feet. By writing the alphabet, you work your feet in all planes of movement and hence address all thirty some muscles that comprise your ankle foot and toes. The trick with this exercise is to not move much at your knee or hip and focus on only moving your ankle and foot.

The twist on the third exercise is simple. Rather than writing the alphabet, pick an affirmation for the day and write that out with each foot. I have listed a few affirmations below to get started. Just to organize my mind the theme of my affirmations is feet, although I occasionally digress a bit. Affirmations can be as simple as "Just do it" to borrow from Nike or "Most people are about as happy as they make up their minds to be" from the heroic Abe Lincoln. Of course, the longer the affirmation, the more exercise for your feet, so you may want to start with a shorter phrase and work your way up to a longer sentence.

Foot Affirmations:

I have included the author of the quotes when I could find the credits for them. Most I have heard or said so often that I am not sure where they originated—within me or someone else honestly. But regardless, "Imitation is the sincerest form of flattery"—Charles Caleb Colton. So whether the source is identified or not, I would like to thank whomever these quotes came from for having an influence on my life and hopefully yours as well.

- "Put your best foot forward."
- "Jump into life feet first."
- "Slow and steady wins the race."—David Lloyd
- "Beauty is but skin deep."—Sir Thomas Overbury
- "A journey begins with a single step."
- "Put one foot in front of the other."—remember the Christmas Special "Santa Clause is Coming to Town"? I sing that theme song to all my kids (both biological and children of the heart) when I'm teaching them how to walk. That song is a great analogy to life in general when we're trying to persevere through difficult times. Another phrase comes to mind on that theme—
- "One step at a time"

- "Baby steps"—in reference to the fact that we can't change everything at once. Sometimes we can only do little things…which leads me to my favorite quote…
- "Small things done with Great Love"— Mother Theresa

So this little book is my small thing done with great love. Perhaps you have found something herein that has given you useful information, support, inspiration, or just food for thought. The bumper sticker on my car reads: "Change happens at the speed of thought." I sincerely hope this book has helped and will continue to help you bring about positive changes in your life for a happier and healthier body, mind, and spirit. Remember, you are changing everyday really, whether you like it or not. Cellular growth and demise is a constant in our body. However, "Change is inevitable, Growth is optional."

Growth is an active process. Only through growth can we feed the masses, learn to walk by faith rather than by fear, and become the people that God designed us to be. Faith, hope, and love need to be put into action to be felt within yourself and within our world. Saint Francis of Assisi once said to preach the gospel with your life and to use words only when absolutely necessary.

I am not sure whether my words have been necessary for you, but in this case, they have certainly been beneficial for me to bring about personal healing and I thank you for sharing this experience with me. My heartfelt desire is that my book can now help you as it has me to continue growing in body, mind, and spirit through the rest of your beautifully balanced life.

Quick Position Guide to Exercise Sequence

Following is an inclusive list of all the exercises in this book with corresponding page numbers. If one wishes to do a complete program the following is an order that will minimize position changes and page turning. Depending on the number of repetitions and the duration of hold for stretches, this program should take between thirty and forty minutes. A few exercises were repeated in different areas to accommodate those who may want to do just a couple sections at a time. Also, doing just two or three exercises from each position will shorten your workout when you are in a time crunch.

1. Upper Trunk Floating/Legs Crossed
    a. Diphragmatic/Deep Breathing, 44
    b. Shoulder Rolls, 44
    c. Neck Range of Motion, 45

2. Upright Sitting with Good Posture
   a. Triceps Stretch, 53
   b. Hamstring Stretch, 54
   c. Piriformis Stretch, 60
   d. Shoulder Extension Stretch, 61
   e. Isometric triceps, 77
   f. Antigravity triceps, 78
   g. Reverse pushups, 78
3. Reclining—Feet Up on Front Edge of Bathtub or Floor of Tub
   a. Bathtub Bridges, 92
   b. Adductor Sets, 96
   c. Heel Slides, 97
   d. Straight Leg Raise, 98
   e. Quad Sets, 99
   f. Pelvic Tilt, 109
   g. Crunches/ Tummy Tucks, 111
   h. Tucks With a Twist, 112
   i. Sit up Slide, 114
4. Reclining with Head at Front of Tub
   a. Push Pull Slide, 113
5. Reclining–Relaxed Knees Bent—Feet on Floor of Bathtub
   a. Glut Sets, 91
   b. Snow Angels 95
   c. Triceps—Reverse Push-ups, 78
   d. Shoulder Extension Stretch, 61
   e. Isometric External Rotators, 80
   f. Kegels, 109

g. Foot/ankle Exercises, 140
6. On Stomach
    a. Prone Push-ups, 119
    b. Bathtub Plank, 120
    c. Prone Hip Extension, 121
    d. Hamstring Curls, 102
7. Side-lying
    a. Side-lying Sit-ups, 117
    b. Quadriceps Stretch, 116
    c. Clam Shells, 96
8. Upright Sitting with Good Posture
    a. Abductor Sets, 94
    b. Shampoo Shuffle, 75
    c. Bicep Curls, 75
    d. Long Arc Quads, 101
    e. Long Sitting Stretch, 59
    f. Feet Affirmations, 141
9. Facing Out of Bathtub
    a. Sole Sitting Stretch, 55
    b. Side Sitting Stretch, 58
10. Standing
    a. Heel Cord Stretch, 129
    b. Toe-and-Heel Lifts, 130-131
    c. Squats, 131
    d. Stork Stance, 132
    e. Hamstring Curls, 133
    f. Standing Hamstring Stretch, 128